MADDISSON LEE

Breastfeeding for Mummies

A survival guide for the breastfeeding mom

First edition

This book was professionally typeset on Reedsy.
Find out more at reedsy.com

To all the mothers out there, you may feel alone sometimes, but we are always here for each other. It can be hard, but but being a mom is one of the most rewarding journeys we will ever experience. I wouldn't trade single day.

Contents

1

From Clueless to Capable: My Breastfeeding Adventure Begins

I remember that first night home from the hospital like it was yesterday. The house was quiet except for the soft little breaths of my newborn son, and my whispering of the "Gilmore Girls" theme song "Where You Lead" by Carole King to him. It was then at that moment, with that little eight-pound baby boy in my arms that I had an overwhelming realization: my life was never, ever going to be the same again. Hi, I'm Maddisson, and I am a first-time mom to a squishy and very energetic little boy. And let's just say, I had as much experience with breastfeeding as I did with taming lions. Spoiler alert: zero.

I don't have any background in the medical field or experience with breastfeeding, nor had I been around anyone who had breastfed. Breastfeeding has been around since mothers have been birthing children, yet somehow, I felt like I was discovering fire. Society has progressed, and women have found various ways of feeding their babies—from breast to pumping to formula. When I was a baby, I was breastfed for less than six weeks before being put on formula because my mother struggled with inverted nipples. None of my family members were breastfed or breastfed their own children. This experience was brand new to me, and I had to learn through doing. I had the help of hospital nurses, a wonderful lactation consultant whom I saw regularly, and a full community of an online breastfeeding group for mothers.

Breastfeeding was no walk in the park. It was more like a stumble through a dark, twisty forest. I faced many of the common hurdles that mothers encounter and discovered that with perseverance, patience, and the willingness to seek help (and being stubborn of course) made all the difference for myself and my little boy.

This book is not a definitive guide or a one-size-fits-all solution. (It also should not be used to replace any medical advice given by actual medical professionals.) It's meant to be a companion, maybe even a source of comfort, and a practical guide for mothers at any stage of their breastfeeding journey. Whether you are pregnant and considering breastfeeding or in the early days of nursing your newborn, my goal is to offer support and solidarity. I want my readers to know that they are not alone in this experience. But also understand that every single mother and baby are different, and what works for one may not work for another.

I came into motherhood, like most, with little knowledge and many misconceptions. I initially thought breastfeeding was going to be about as fun as a root canal. In the beginning my nipples were sore, my baby didn't latch properly, and there were countless moments when doubt and exhaustion overwhelmed me. Yet, amidst the chaos, there were many moments of deep connection, satisfaction, and the profound realization that I was providing my baby with the best nourishment and comfort that only I could give.

In the chapters that follow, I will take you through the various stages of my journey. From the initial decision to breastfeed, through the early days of learning and adapting, to the more complex challenges of pumping and balancing life, and finally, to the bittersweet decision of weaning. Along the way, I'll share practical tips, personal anecdotes, and the wisdom I've gained from both my own experiences and the experiences of others.

Let's embark on this milk-filled adventure together!

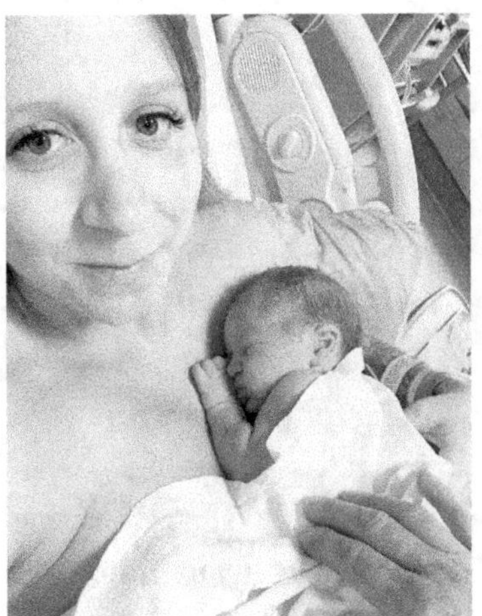 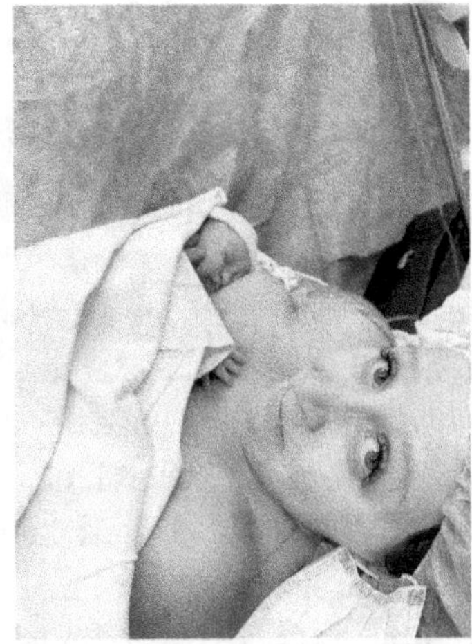

My son and I the day he was born

2

Pregnancy, Panic, and Pumping Plans

I was thirty-four years old when I found out I was pregnant, and my emotions were like a rollercoaster in a hurricane. I'd always dreamed of having my own family, but my visions never included a perfect wedding (though I am happily married)—just babies. Lots of squishy, adorable babies.

My husband and I had been planning for this baby for years. I'd been on birth control for eighteen and a half years, so when we finally decided to start planning more seriously, it was time for me to come off "The Pill". With the help of my naturopath it took almost two years for my hormones to play nice again. Once my hormones were more balanced and accommodating to a woman wanting to conceive, we consulted our family physician to make sure we were good to go.

Our doctor, ever the bearer of terrifying news, informed us that it takes the average couple sixteen months to get pregnant and that most women go through about three miscarriages. (Now, I don't know how much of this is true or just here-say as I did not have the stomach to go home and research such things). To say I left that appointment feeling like I'd been hit by a truck would be an understatement. I was reeling, wondering why it had to be so difficult and why it would take so long with such traumatizing steps. And to top it off, I was labeled as having a "geriatric pregnancy." Lovely. But my husband, the eternal optimist, told me to take it with a grain of salt. He reminded me that doctors must consider all possibilities and that stressing out wouldn't help.

There is a First for Everything

Armed with an ovulation test kit, we eagerly began trying for a baby. Miraculously, it worked on the first go! When my period didn't show up, I took a pregnancy test and nearly fainted when it was positive. I remember holding that little stick, watching the second line appear, and feeling a wave of disbelief wash over me. I decided to wait a week before telling my husband, wanting to surprise him in a special way.

During that week, I could hardly contain my excitement and nervousness. I handmade a little baby onesie with the words "Just in time for hunting season" because my husband is outdoorsy and our baby was due in the fall, right during hunting season. When the day finally came to share the news, I handed him both the onesie and the positive pregnancy test. He looked at both, his face slowly transforming from confusion to sheer joy. He was over the moon excited, literally jumping for joy! I burst into tears the moment I told him, and we both stood there, holding each other, filled with happiness and excitement.

Suddenly, I had a million decisions to make, each one more significant than the last. We spent the rest of the day in a daze, alternating between bouts of joyous laughter and moments of quiet contemplation. Breastfeeding hadn't even crossed my mind at this point. We were just basking in the reality of our little miracle, imagining what the future would hold for our growing family.

As my pregnancy progressed, I waded through the sea of opinions on how to feed my baby. Every gathering with friends and family and casual conversation seemed to come with un-solicited advice. Some swore by breastfeeding, painting it as the ultimate bonding experience and a health booster for both mom and baby. Others sang the praises of formula, emphasizing its convenience and how it allowed other family members to participate in feeding.

Financially, formula was out for us, but breastfeeding sounded like a nightmare. I vividly remember an acquaintance at work recounting her horror stories about sore nipples, endless leaks, and sheer exhaustion. "Yikes," I thought. The more I heard, the more overwhelmed I felt. Each story added to my anxiety, making me question my ability to handle what was coming.

In quieter moments, my husband and I would sit together, discussing our options and trying to find a path that felt right for us. He was incredibly supportive, reminding me that whatever decision we made, it would be the best one for our family. His calm reassurance was a beacon of hope amidst the storm of opinions and fears swirling in my mind.

Through it all, I tried to focus on the excitement of becoming a mother, reminding myself that millions of women had navigated these waters before me. I knew that, somehow, we would find our way too.

Colostrum Surprise

Around the four-month mark in my pregnancy, I noticed a yellow, oozy substance on my nipples while showering. Panic mode activated! I've never had anything come from my nipples before! I yelled for my husband to come and see just to make sure I wasn't imagining things. He took one look, scrunched up his face, and muttered, "Ew!" before fleeing the bathroom. Men, right?

I checked with my OB-GYN, who explained that my breasts were gearing up for milk production and the yellow stuff was called colostrum. I decided then that I would not breastfeed, I would strictly pump and bottle-feed. The idea of breastfeeding made me feel a little queasy.

Despite the advice from well-meaning friends and family who gifted me breastfeeding videos and books, I couldn't bring myself to watch or read them. The only thing I read was the few pages from "What to Expect When You're Expecting" on breastfeeding. As my due date approached, I felt increasingly nervous and unprepared.

At a much later OB appointment, I was told to express colostrum and given a video link. Watching other women express milk scared me senseless, and I worried I'd do it wrong and hurt myself.

I was lucky to secure an appointment at a top-notch lactation clinic four days before my scheduled C-section. My husband came with me and joined me in the exam room, fiddling with every medical device he could get his hands on—typical.

The room was softly lit, and the doctor's calm presence put me at ease. She had me unclip my nursing tank and with icy cold hands, gently squeezed my breasts, showing me how to express milk. To my relief, it didn't hurt at all! What was I so afraid of? I left that appointment feeling much more confident than before.

Operation Baby Day

In the days leading up to the birth, I re-read sections of my pregnancy. Everything pointed to breast milk being packed with essential nutrients and antibodies. The idea of skin-to-skin bonding and reducing the risk of illnesses for both of us sealed the deal. I still wouldn't feed directly from my breasts, but I was ready to pump and bottle-feed.

Finally, the big day arrived. "Baby Day," as my husband and I referred to it, was here. We drove to the hospital in the early morning, the car ride filled with a nervous excitement. The hospital staff were wonderful, guiding us through each step with warmth and reassurance. The operating room was a blur of cool, sterile smells and the hum of machines. My heart raced with a mix of fear and excitement as I was prepped for the C-section. My husband held my hand, his presence a calming anchor in the midst of the medical whirlwind.

When they held up my squishy little boy, his cries filled the room, and my heart exploded with love. Tears streamed down my face as they placed him on my chest. His tiny body fit perfectly in my arms, and he immediately started rooting for the breast like a tiny, hungry dinosaur. It was a surreal and beautiful moment, one that I will treasure forever.

Despite my plans to pump only, I let him latch on. Ouch! It wasn't at all what I had expected, but it felt incredibly natural. His little mouth latched onto my breast, and though the sensation was new and a bit uncomfortable, it also felt right. In that moment, I knew I was made to breastfeed my son. The initial pain gave way to a profound sense of connection and purpose.

Beginning the Journey

And so, our breastfeeding journey began, filled with challenges and triumphs. Each step brought us closer together, and

I discovered strengths within myself I never knew existed. The days and nights blurred together as we navigated the learning curve of breastfeeding. There were moments of doubt and exhaustion, but also moments of pure joy and deep bonding.

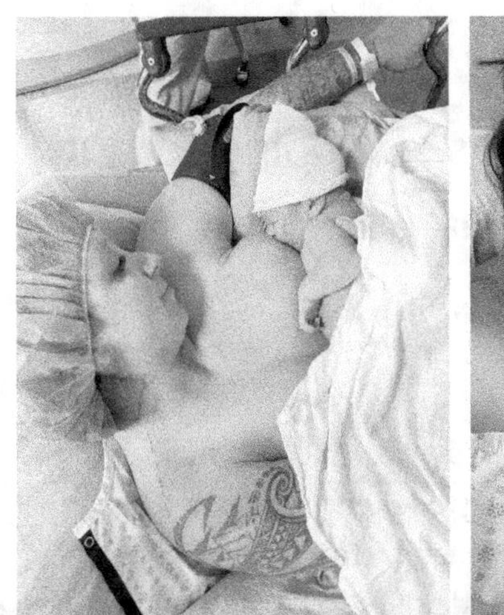
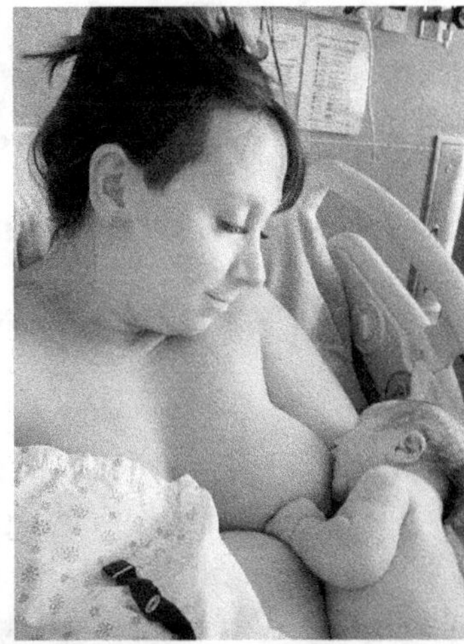

(Left) The very moment my son latched for the first time (Right) In awe watching my son nurse

3

Gear Up, Mummies! Prepping for the Breastfeeding Adventure

When I had decided to pump and feed my baby with breast milk, finding the right breast pump became a priority. Little did I know, this decision would lead me into the wild and wacky world of breastfeeding accessories too. Some of these gadgets were lifesavers, while others I found un-necessary. Let me take you on a tour of my treasure trove of breastfeeding gear, complete with some laughs along the way.

- **Breast Pump:** Even if you plan to exclusively breastfeed directly from the breast, having a breast pump is like having a magic wand. I chose an electric double pump for efficiency. After extensive research (more like late-night Google rabbit holes), I settled on one that offered more portability. I didn't want to be tied to an electrical outlet every time I needed to use it, and I certainly didn't want to lug around a behemoth of a pump. This nifty gadget was a game-changer for increasing my milk supply and relieving engorgement. Pro tip: get a second set of breast shields and flange inserts.

Trust me, when you're up at 3 AM, the last thing you want to do is wash pump parts. Just grab the spare set and keep the milk flowing!

- **Breast Pads**: Disposable or reusable breast pads were essential for preventing leaks in the early days. The reusable ones were too bulky and the thought of washing them constantly made me want to cry. Disposable ones, on the other hand, were a lifesaver. They soaked up the leaks and saved me from many embarrassing moments. I always kept a few in my pumping kit and in the diaper bag so I'd have them whenever I needed.

- **Breast Therapy Hot & Cold Packs**: These reusable round gel packs can be frozen or heated to provide hot or cold relief for tender, overworked breasts. They're also great for blocked ducts or mastitis. I even used them for my little guy's upset tummy, they were the perfect size, and the soft covers ensured they weren't too hot against his skin.

- **Flange Inserts**: Breast shields are not a one-size-fits-all and are often too large for most women. Even if your breasts doubled in size like mine did! But luckily, they make small silicone inserts, referred too as "Flange Inserts", which are designed to improve comfort and fit. I had no idea that these even existed, and I sure wish I did before I had started using my pump! One night, the first week home with my son, while attempting to pump hands-free and waiting for dinner to warm in the microwave, I felt a warm, wet sensation soaking through my socks. I looked down to see a stream of breast milk running down my stomach, soaking my pants, and pooling on the kitchen floor. My precious 'liquid gold' was wasted all over the floor! I was devastated and pretty frustrated. Thankfully, my lactation consultant told me that nipples, like snowflakes, come in all shapes and sizes. She introduced me to flange inserts, and voilà! No more spilled milk.

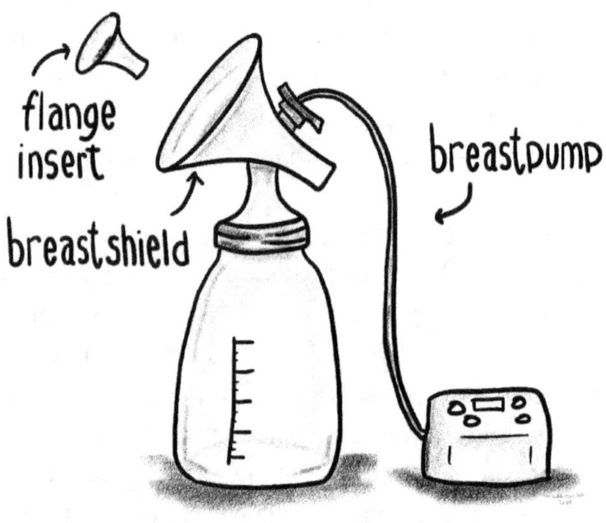

A simple drawing I made to show the flanges, breast shield and pump

- **Nipple Cream:** I tried three different lanolin-based nipple creams from my local store. While they might work for some, they didn't help me. My lactation consultant prescribed a cream with antifungal and ibuprofen properties, which was a lifesaver for my sore nipples in those early days.
- **Nipple Shields:** Nipple shields are thin, flexible silicone or

rubber covers designed to fit over the nipple and areola during breastfeeding. They help with various issues, including latching problems and sore nipples. I didn't need them for feeding, but they were a godsend for preventing irritation from bed sheets and blankets during those first sore, raw days.

- **Nursing Bras and Tops:** Nursing bras were not my friends. They were too constricting and caused blocked ducts. Instead, I fell in love with nursing tanks. They were comfortable, easy to open, and made public breastfeeding a breeze. I bought a set around seven months pregnant when my pre-pregnancy bras no longer fit, and they've been a staple in my wardrobe ever since. I also invested in some nursing sweaters that had concealed zippers over each breast, and they allowed easy access while also remaining discreet.

- **Nursing Cover:** While not essential, a nursing cover provided me with added privacy when breastfeeding in public. There is a strap/loop to go around the back of your neck (like an apron) to keep it in place and a wire along the top edge that forms a hoop, allowing you the ability to see the baby feeding while remaining covered.

- **Nursing Pillow:** A good nursing pillow made positioning my baby comfortable and reduced strain on my back and arms. This was especially helpful with a larger baby. Buy two. One for the nursery and one for your common area. You will thank me later.

- **Storage Bags:** Breast milk storage bags allowed me to freeze and store expressed milk safely and neatly. I used different brands, but I found that the measurements on the bags were inaccurate on all of them. Using a measuring cup before pouring into the storage bag helped me keep track of the correct amounts.

- **Silver Nipple Cups**: These small, dome-shaped cups made from pure silver or silver-plated materials are designed to soothe and heal sore, cracked, or damaged nipples. I had them in my breast pump bag but found they kept my nipples too moist and sticky. They're popular among many mothers, so you might find they work for you.

- **At-Home Nursing Station**: Creating a comfortable breast-feeding environment at home was a key step. I set up a dedicated nursing station in my living room with a comfy chair, good lighting, and all my supplies within arm's reach. I also had a station next to my bed for nighttime feeds. Having these setups made nursing sessions more relaxed and enjoyable and made it so I didn't have to disturb the baby by getting up constantly. Keeping a water bottle and healthy snacks nearby helped me stay hydrated and nourished too, as breastfeeding can be physically demanding.

- **Ready-Made Snacks & Meals:** Before my son arrived, I naively believed I'd have plenty of free time. Looking back, I wish I had done more food preparation for myself and my family. Most of my resting time was spent nursing, snuggling, recovering, and sleeping. I was unprepared for the intense hunger that accompanied breastfeeding. Filling the fridge and pantry with quick, grab-and-go snacks and high-protein options proved essential. Packing a small lunch bag with a water bottle and healthy snacks like peanut butter sandwiches, trail mix, cheese sticks, apple slices, granola bars, and lactation cookies allowed me to stay nourished as I moved from room to room. The convenience of having these snacks within reach made a significant difference in my ability to care for my newborn. Particularly while recovering from a C-section.

Overall, preparing for breastfeeding before bringing home the baby was quite the process. My husband used to joke that I was "being clucky," describing the "nesting phase" we all go through before a baby is born. It was a rewarding and comforting process. And who doesn't love shopping, organizing, and prepping?

Gathering the right supplies and setting up a comfortable space made me feel more confident and ready to embark on my breastfeeding journey. As you prepare for your own journey, remember that while preparation is important, flexibility and patience are key. Every mother's experience is unique, and what matters most is finding what works best for you and your baby. For example, different opinions exist on what nursing chair is best. Many mothers prefer a glider-type rocking chair, but I went with a "Lazy Boy" design. It rocked, glided, and reclined when needed and I found that for the first few weeks I spent almost all my time in it. Comfort was key.

So, gear up, mummies! You've got this!

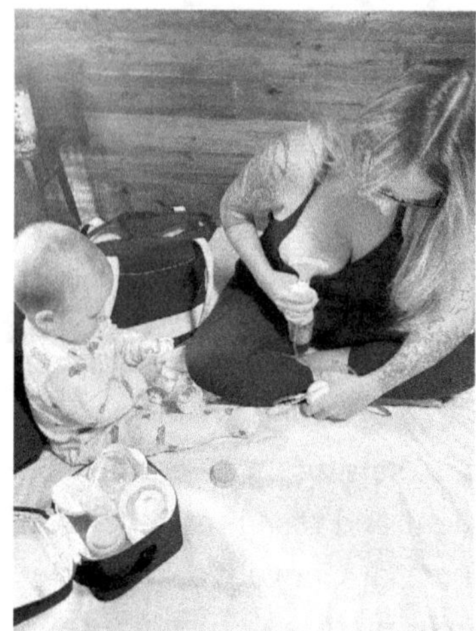 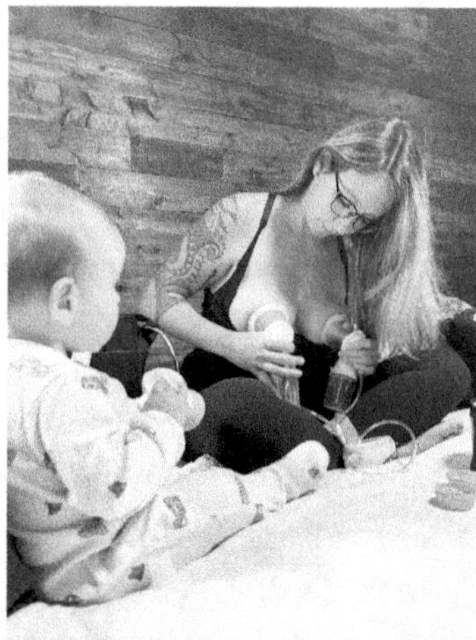

(Left) Pumping a single breast (Right) Pumping both breasts simultaneously

4

Surviving the First Feeds: Tales from the Trenches

The first moments of breastfeeding often occur in the hospital, right after birth. My experience was both overwhelming and enlightening. The support from the hospital staff, particularly the nurses, was invaluable. Not only did they respect my wishes about not wanting to formula feed, but they also encouraged nursing. They guided me through the initial latch, helped me position my baby in different ways, and reassured me when things didn't go perfectly. During my three-day stay, I received advice and tips from several nurses, each offering unique insights to help me navigate this new adventure as a first-time mom. I was very fortunate as I've heard many stories about mothers being pressured into formula and bottle feeding right from birth.

Skin-to-Skin Magic

Skin-to-skin contact played a magical role in those early hours and days. It was essential not only for bonding but also for stimulating milk production. It was incredible to see that when my baby was placed against my chest for the first time, he immediately started going for the breast like he had a built-in GPS. I spent as much time as possible holding him against me while I was in the hospital, letting him familiarize himself with me and me with him. After spending the better part of a year feeling him grow and move inside my belly, the empty, aching feeling of his absence was overwhelming. Holding him helped ease that transition. And when that squishy little baby wasn't lying directly on me, he was always within sight and arm's reach.

Once we got home, the skin-to-skin struggle was real. My husband, bless him, insisted that our son needed to learn how to self-soothe. I felt guilty whenever I was holding and snuggling my son, yet it was the only thing I wanted to do every moment of every day. My husband would see me with our son on my chest and would tell me that he needed some time in his rocking chair to get used to being alone. He wasn't trying to be negative; he just didn't want our son to end up like his friends' kids who couldn't be set down or still slept in their parents' bed as teenagers. I'll be honest, I resented him for making me feel this way, and I believe it worsened my postpartum depression. Sometimes I would reluctantly set my son down and I would see my husband pick him up to snuggle, and it upset me further, bringing to the surface postpartum rage. The urge to snatch that little baby from his arms was overwhelming! But! I didn't act on harsh feelings, but the feelings were something I had never experienced before. While it's important for fathers to bond with their babies, I couldn't help feeling selfish and not wanting to share my son with anyone. Even him.

Thankfully, my mother was there to advocate for me and my little guy. She would often say out loud that a newborn baby, only days old, is much too young to have to learn to self-soothe. During our follow-up appointments, the doctors also reassured me that skin-to-skin was one of the greatest gifts I could give my son. It helps babies regulate their body temperature and emotions and helps mothers regulate their hormones and deepen the bond with the tiny human they spent over nine months growing inside them. The days and weeks following my sons birth I could see how quickly time was passing. People always said that "time flies" but it wasn't until becoming a mother myself that I truly understood just how fast. I felt like I needed to hold him every chance I could because I was worried that if I didn't, I'd regret it and the moments would be gone forever. I regret not holding him more as a newborn baby. I regret not being more in the moment with him during those newborn days.

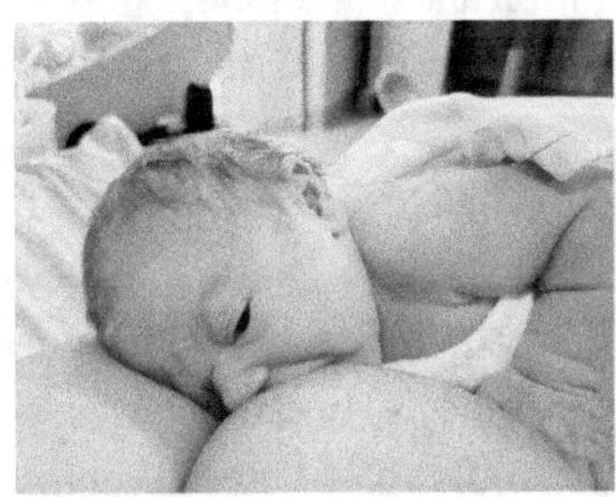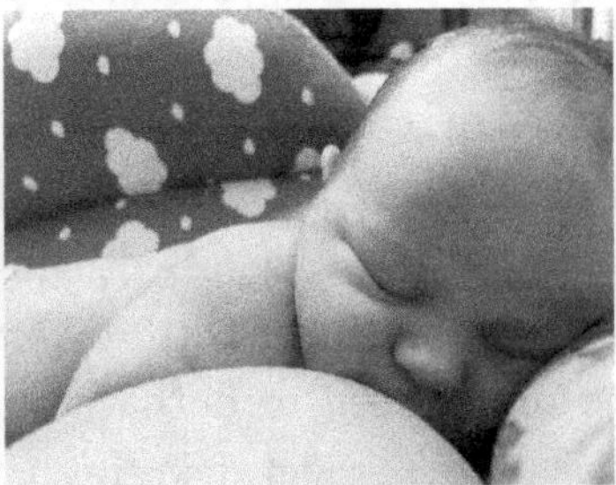

(Left) Nursing skin-to-skin (Right) A skin-to-skin nap, post feed

Latch, Unlatch, Repeat

Latching issues were particularly challenging at first. Despite the wealth of knowledge and support from the hospital nurses, it wasn't until our second day there that I realized I was latching the baby incorrectly. One nurse, observing us, pointed out that he was only suckling on the tip of the nipple and not fully around it and the areola, and provided further guidance. This moment highlighted the importance of continuous learning and support in the early days of breastfeeding. When the baby is latched but needs to be corrected (which happens often in the beginning), she showed me a nifty trick: put your finger into their mouth between the gums to force them to open their mouth and break away from the nipple. Unlatch, relatch, repeat. It felt like a never-ending dance routine.

The Painful Truth

Before I learned how to correct his latch, I often dreaded bringing the baby to my breasts. They were raw and sore, and the pain was sharp and unforgettable, like a constant reminder of our struggle. Each time he latched, I braced myself for the discomfort, feeling a mix of frustration and helplessness. It was like my nipples were auditioning for a horror movie, and they nailed the role of "Victim #1."

Seeing me wince when the baby latched to feed, my husband, bless his heart, suggested giving my breasts a break and instead offering the baby a bottle of formula. Though I had decided not to formula feed, we did have a can at home just in case. However, just the thought of giving my baby formula upset me to the point of tears. I felt like resorting to formula meant I was failing and doing something wrong. My initial goal was to breastfeed to six months, and I refused to give in and give up just because I was sore, tired and found it difficult. I was adamant that the baby and I would figure it all out. Patience was certainly a must. Over time, as my baby and I became more in sync, breastfeeding became easier and more comfortable. It was like we finally learned the choreography to our breastfeeding dance, and the pain started to fade like a distant memory.

The Support Squad

One of the most important aspects of those early days was the support system around me. My husband, family, and friends played critical roles in providing emotional and practical support. My mom came to stay with me for the first three weeks after we brought the baby home. She was there to help me get to and from doctor's appointments and was a lifesaver the evenings, allowing me three to four consecutive hours of uninterrupted sleep. She also relished in this time with her firstborn grandson. My husband, even working a full-time day job, took it upon himself to get up with me each night to help me with diaper changes and nursing until I was comfortable enough to take it on myself. Having a c-section delivery meant that I was limited on what I could do for a couple of weeks, and he was there alongside my mother helping me with whatever I or the baby needed. My husband often reminded me, "this is all temporary," meaning that although everything seemed daunting in the moment, these challenges would soon pass. His words became a comforting mantra, helping me stay patient and focused on the progress we were making. He was my rock, supporting me through the tough nights and celebrating the small victories. He would change the baby, bring me snacks and water while I nursed, and was always ready with a word of encouragement or a funny story to lift my spirits. We became a team, united in our love for our son and our determination to give him the best start in life.

Diaper Disasters

I can remember (and still laugh about it to this day) the very first diaper change I ever did. It was very early in the morning; the room was dark, and I was delirious from lack of sleep. The diaper change seemed more difficult than it should have been at the time, but I did not give it much thought in that moment. When we got up in the morning to do another diaper change, we found that I had, in fact, put the baby's diaper on backwards! No wonder I couldn't find the tabs! It made for a good laugh between myself, my mother, and my husband.

One messy side of feeding babies that people don't talk about (and should!) is that breastfed babies don't have smelly poops. They can also go up to fourteen days without a bowel movement! Fourteen days?! Yikes. Could you imagine? The consistency of the poop stayed the same until we started solids a few months later and it was an easy way to determine if anything was ever off with the baby or if he were ill. You want to talk about smelly poops? My goodness, with the introduction of solids, just you wait! I've also heard that formula-fed babies make for some smelly little beings too. I'm grateful that we didn't have to experience those messy diapers! Pee yew.

From Gas to Giggles

While the diaper mishap provided a good laugh, other challenges were less amusing. When my son was around three to four weeks old, we faced a new hurdle—our little guy was struggling with consistent discomfort and gas. This led us to our next big lesson. We were initially told that we did not ever have to worry about him overfeeding on breast milk. Babies that nurse only consume what they need and instinctively know when to stop. However, we learned the hard way that this wasn't entirely true.

A visit to our Lactation Consultant's office for a weighted feed revealed that he was taking in about 80-90ml more than he should have during a feed. That was almost double the amount that his stomach could hold and digest. This discovery prompted our consultant to adjust our routine, suggesting we nurse from one breast at a time only and stop offering both breasts to him each time we nursed. After about four to five days, the difference was noticeable. My son was a much happier little guy, no longer suffering from an upset stomach and excess gas.

One morning I was nursing my son quietly in his room, getting him fed and ready to lay down for a nap in his crib. I knew to wait a few extra minutes after he'd fallen asleep before moving him to lay in his bed and tiptoe out of the room. This one time I had only just started to get up from the rocking chair and he immediately started to cry. It was so funny to me because though he was sound asleep, he still knew what I was planning to do. The separation anxiety phase, around the nine-to-ten-month age, was a challenge all on its own. Well, I sat back down quietly, and he fell back to sleep in an instant. I couldn't help but laugh! I don't know what I found so funny in that moment, but I laughed hard. My son peaked open one eye to look up at me and when he saw me laughing, he burst out laughing too! We must've sat there for another five minutes just laughing at each other! The nap was ruined, but the moment brought tears to my eyes. Seeing a happy baby, not experiencing any discomfort and relishing in the bonding just filled my heart.

Which Position?

With the help of hospital nurses and our Lactation Consultant, I learned that using the right position can make a significant difference in comfort and effectiveness. Here are some common positions that I learned about and a couple I found helpful:

- **Cradle Hold:** This classic position involves holding the baby across your lap, supporting their head with the crook of your arm. It's great for newborns and allows for close eye contact.

- **Cross-Cradle Hold**: Similar to the cradle hold, but with the baby's head supported by the opposite arm. This position provides more control over the baby's head and is useful for achieving a good latch. This became one of our go-to positions as my baby grew and got heavier, accounting for more than half of our feeding sessions.

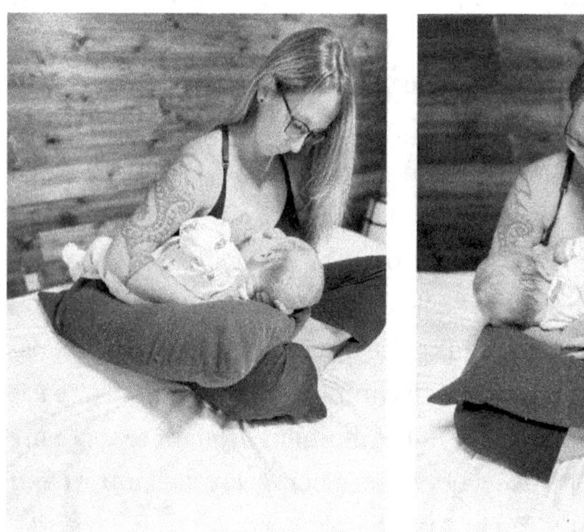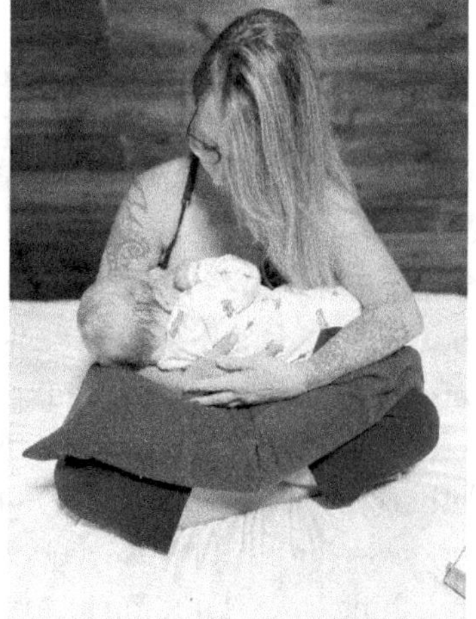

(Left) Nursing in the "Football Hold" (Right) Nursing in the "Cross-cradle Hold"

- **Football Hold**: Holding the baby at your side, under your arm like a football, can be particularly useful for mothers recovering from a C-section or for those with larger breasts. This position allows you to see the baby's latch more clearly.

We used this primarily for the first 4-6 weeks because it provided the best latch and kept the weight off my incision site.

- **Side-Lying Position:** Lying on your side with the baby facing you is a comfortable position for nighttime feedings or when you need to rest. It allows both mother and baby to relax during feeding. This was another favorite for us, especially during those early morning wake-ups or middle of the night comfort sessions when I was just too tired to pull myself out of bed.

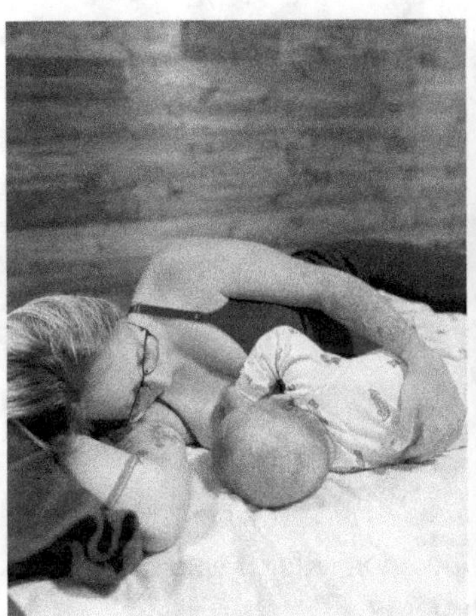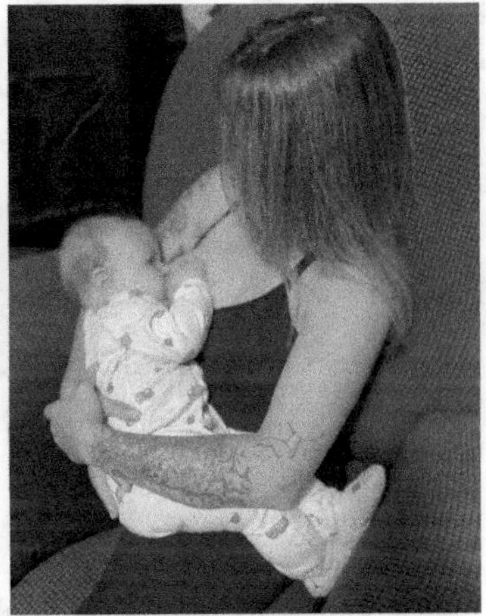

(Left) Nursing in the "Side-lying" position (Right) Nursing in the "Cradle" hold

- **Laid-Back Position**: Also known as biological nurturing, this position involves reclining comfortably with the baby lying on your chest. Gravity helps with the latch, and it's particularly good for encouraging skin-to-skin contact. As an over supplier, I found this position useful when my milk flow was too strong for my baby to manage on his own.

By trying out different positions, we found what worked best for us and made the feeding experience more enjoyable and comfortable. Every baby is different, so don't be afraid to experiment until you find what works best for you.

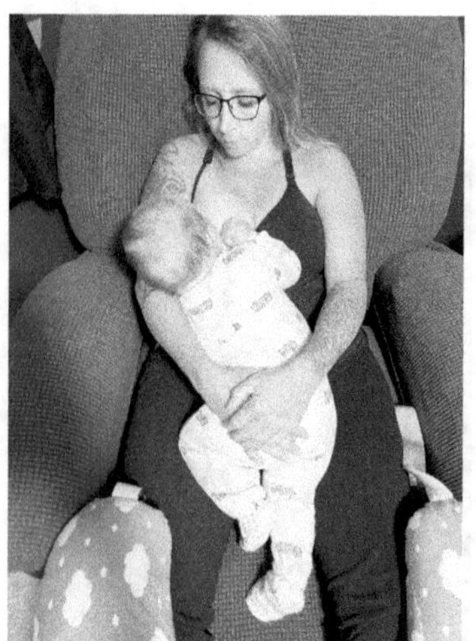
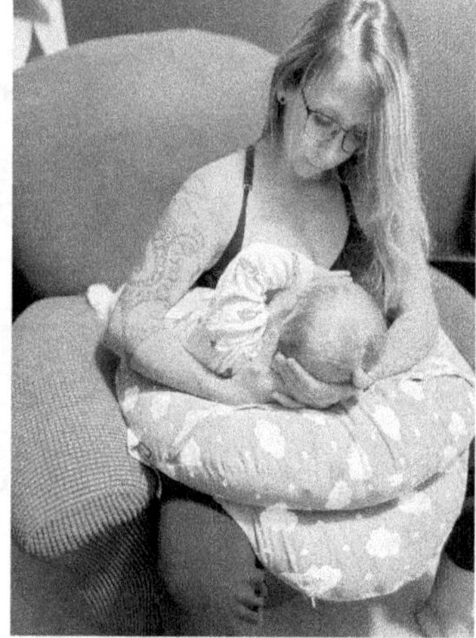

(Left) Nursing in the "Laid Back" position (Right) Nursing in the "Football Hold"

5

Boobie Battles: Tackling Common Breastfeeding Problems

I'd heard of some of the common issues of nursing before I started my journey, and they were originally what made me reluctant to choose this over formula. Here are the common issues among most mothers, in no particular order:

Sore nipples: Ah yes! sore and cracked nipples—the joy that every nursing mother gets to experience. Oh, my word. I had no idea how raw, cracked, and painful they could be! I had bought multiple over-the-counter lanolin nipple creams but found that they didn't really help me. I wish that I had known from the start that nursing shouldn't be painful. I honestly didn't know what to think of this feeling. I had just assumed that this was part of the process and didn't know I been doing anything incorrectly. There should be a pulling feeling, but not a painful pull.

I have never had to get into the shower and cover up my breasts with my arm or hands before this time in my life because even something as relaxing as a warm shower was enough to irritate my poor nipples. I was fortunate to have my Lactation

Consultant prescribe a cream to use in place of the store-bought ones. After only a few days of regular application my nipples were no longer raw, cracked or blistered. Boy what a life saver that cream was!

I also learned that one of the best remedies for sore and cracked nipples is your very own breast milk! Who knew I had a natural pharmacy on tap? In between cream applications, I would express a drop or two of breast milk and leave it on the nipple to dry naturally. Some mothers choose to wear silver nipple cups. I tried them briefly, but they weren't for me. Besides, who needs bling on their boobs?

Latching: A proper latch is vital for effective feeding and preventing nipple pain. I can't stress this enough. It's very important that the baby's mouth be wide open before latching. Think of it as a baby bird trying to eat—a wide, eager mouth. A good latch involves your baby taking in a good portion of the areola (not just the nipple) into their mouth. It should be comfortable for you, with minimal discomfort or pain. Positioning my son correctly, with his body facing mine, his head slightly tilted back with his chin touching and his little nose unobstructed so he could continue to breathe made all the difference. If a baby's latch is too shallow, they will only suck the nipple and not the breast itself, and by sucking on the nipple only, it can cause pain and trauma to the nipple and surrounding area.

If the baby's latch is too big, they will suck in air with each pull, causing an upset stomach and a gassy, uncomfortable baby. Nothing says "fun night" like a gassy baby. It was not only about making it a habit for the baby to latch properly, but it was also about making it a habit for me to watch and inspect his latch at every feed. An ineffective latch can cause milk supply concerns as the breasts may not be adequately stimulated to produce milk.

During the first couple of days of nursing, because the latch was too shallow, both nipples had blistered and bled. It caused severe pain to the nipples themselves but also to the surrounding breast tissue. I was getting these electric shock-type feelings throughout the breast at completely random times during the day and night. The lactation consultant referred to it as vasospasms. It was like my breasts were trying out for a horror movie. She taught us how to recognize a correct and an incorrect latch and recommended that I use cold ice packs after a feed for a couple of weeks until the discomfort subsided.

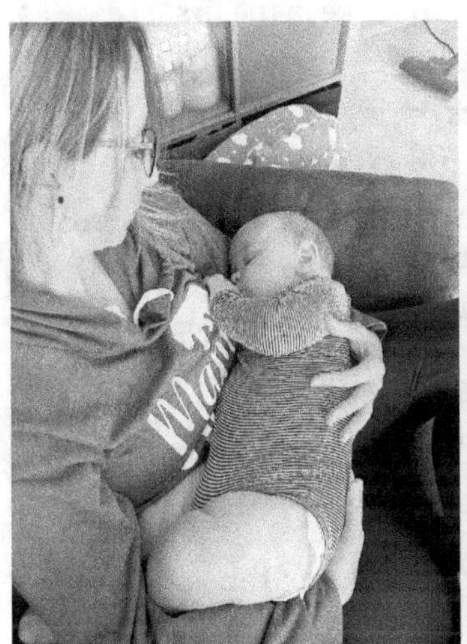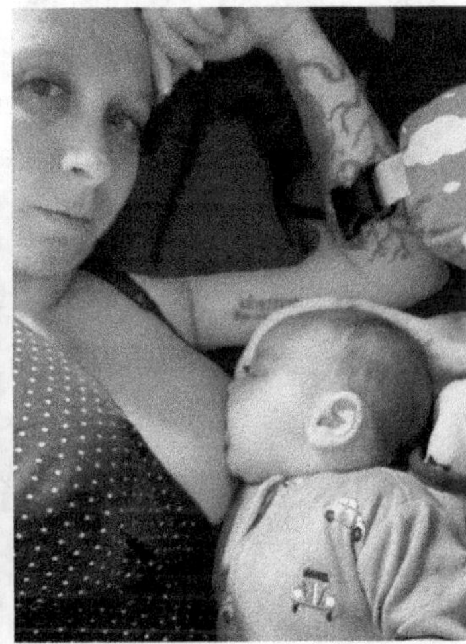

(Left) Replacing a feed with snuggles, a common practice as we started to wean (Right) A tired mum feeding her son in the "side lying" position

Blocked Ducts and Mastitis: Blocked ducts and mastitis, the dynamic duo no one asked for, can crash your nursing party at any time. A blocked duct is like a traffic jam in your boob's milk highway. Milk ducts carry the good stuff from the glands to the nipple, but when one gets blocked, it's like having a stubborn pothole. This can lead to a tender lump that grows slower than a bad mood on a Monday morning, usually forming on one side of the breast. You might notice pink or red skin over the tender area, warmth, and shooting pains that make you wish you could swap your boob for a less problematic one.

Mastitis, on the other hand, is an infection that can turn your breast into a war zone. It's like your breast has caught a nasty cold, but it's no ordinary cold—it's one that needs antibiotics to clear up. Mastitis is most likely to strike in the first six weeks, but it can surprise you anytime during your journey.

I experienced two blocked ducts during my nursing escapades. Luckily, neither turned into mastitis. The first time, I became a self-diagnosed, Google doctor. The pain was so intense I couldn't hold my baby against my body on the affected side. Warm compresses, massages, and cold packs became my new best friends. I made sure to feed the baby frequently on that side to clear the blockage. I kept a wary eye out for mastitis symptoms like fever and chills, but thankfully, after a few hours, the pain subsided.

The second time, I was smarter and booked an appointment with my lactation consultant. She confirmed my self-diagnosis (yay, me!) and reminded me to watch for a fever. She also recommended I take sunflower lecithin regularly to prevent future blockages. The lecithin was like putting a "No Parking" sign on my milk ducts.

There are a few things that a mother can do to prevent and help if they ever experience a blocked duct or mastitis:

- Alternate applying hot and cold compresses.
- Massage the breast from the outer edges towards the nipple.
- Pump or feed regularly every couple of hours to empty.
- Use vibration on the breast using an electric toothbrush.
- Wear looser fitting clothing or bras. Too much pressure can increase the risk of clogs.
- Take Lecithin (sunflower or soy) daily. But ensure to check with your doctor first.

Cluster Feeding: Cluster feeding is a term that could easily be mistaken for a group activity, but it's just your baby's way of turning you into an all-you-can-eat buffet. Instead of feeding every 2-3 hours, your little one might want to nurse every thirty minutes to an hour, especially during the late afternoon or evening—right when you'd prefer to be winding down. It's like they know when you're trying to watch your favorite show and decide that's the perfect time for extra snacks.

At first, identifying these feeding frenzies was like trying to predict the weather. It messed with our developing routine and left me feeling like a dairy cow on overdrive. My well-meaning support system often questioned why he wanted to feed so often, sometimes suggesting he couldn't possibly be hungry again. Explaining that this phase was temporary, and part of his growth spurt development was a challenge. All I could do was make sure I ate more and stayed extra hydrated to keep up with his demands.

Engorgement: Engorgement is another delightful surprise, where your breasts feel like they're about to explode. This happens when your body produces more milk than your breasts can hold, causing them to feel like overfilled water balloons. It's common in the early days when your milk first comes in, turning your boobs into painful, throbbing lumps of milk and misery.

Engorgement can make it hard for your baby to latch and can lead to blocked ducts and mastitis if not managed. It can be caused by not feeding often enough, poor latch, or even wearing constrictive bras or tops. Here's how to deal with this overabundance of milk:

- Take a warm shower and hand express.
- Use a warm compress briefly on the breasts before feeding to help the milk flow.
- Use a cold compress after a feeding to help relieve pain and reduce swelling.
- Some moms swear by frozen cabbage leaves in their bras—who knew a veggie could double as a remedy?
- Take an anti-inflammatory pain reliever (be sure to talk to your doctor about this first).
- Wear loose fitting clothing.
- Be patient and try not to stress—easier said than done, I know.

I dealt with engorgement frequently within the first year because my body produced more milk than my "Boobie Barnacle," as my husband and I affectionately called him, could consume. My lactation consultant noted that my breasts could hold a larger volume of milk than the average nursing mother's. To help regulate my supply, we switched to a new routine of feeding from one side for a two-hour window before switching to the other side. I was also prescribed medication and supplements to help lower my supply so I wouldn't wake up engorged in the night. Balancing supply and demand were a delicate dance, but with some tweaks, we found our groove.

Excessive Sweating and Odor: During breastfeeding, the body undergoes significant hormonal changes that can affect the way it regulates temperature and sweat production. The increased levels of prolactin and oxytocin, hormones essential for milk production and bonding, can also stimulate the sweat glands. Additionally, the body's metabolism is working harder to produce milk, which can increase body heat and lead to more sweating. This is the body's natural way of cooling down and maintaining a stable internal temperature.

In the first few months postpartum, it wasn't just a light perspiration; it was a full-blown sweat fest that left me feeling sticky and uncomfortable most of the time. It also left me feeling embarrassed when I'd sweat enough for it to show through my clothing. I was self-conscious about going near my husband because I worried he would notice the odor and run for the hills. Though he said he never noticed at all, he may have just been nice to spare my feelings.

From the moment I woke up to the end of the day, I was changing my clothes multiple times and sometimes even showering 2-3 times a day. No matter how often I washed, I couldn't escape the smell. For me, it was like an endless waft of tacos clinging to my skin. Other mothers I spoke to reported smelling like onions. It was a strange and disconcerting experience, adding another layer of stress to the already challenging postpartum period.

On warmer days, the skin-to-skin contact while breastfeeding caused heat rashes to develop on my arms and chest. The doctor advised me to use hydrocortisone cream topically to help keep myself more comfortable. Sometimes, I would have to place a receiving blanket between us to prevent the sweating and reduce the irritation. Imagine trying to explain to a tiny, hungry human that the blanket was necessary to prevent mummy from melting – it was quite the juggling act!

I quickly learned that my usual hygiene routine wasn't going to cut it. I started using antibacterial soap to wash under my arms, hoping to combat the odor more effectively. Additionally, I had to switch to an aluminum-free men's deodorant because women's deodorant just couldn't keep up with the intensity of my postpartum perspiration. The men's deodorant provided better protection, helping me feel a bit more confident and less self-conscious about the smell.

This period of excessive sweating lasted for about 3-4 months, gradually tapering off as my body adjusted to its new hormonal balance.

Illness: It's not uncommon for a mother to fall ill and get sick, and it's amazing how life doesn't stop just because you've got the sniffles. The good news? You don't need to stop nursing when you're sick. In fact, your body becomes a little antibody factory, passing on the immune-boosting benefits to your baby. Just be sure to wash your hands like you're about to perform surgery and wear a mask if necessary.

Low Milk Supply: Low milk supply is a common worry among mothers, and I was no exception. I feared I was running a milk drought. It turns out, it could take two to three days for your milk to come in after delivery, sometimes longer if you had a C-section. In my first week home, I was obsessed with how much I was producing, so I started pumping between feeds. Little did I know, I was setting myself up to become an over-supplier.

I was initially thrilled to pump 1 ounce, and over the moon

when I hit 3 ounces. What I didn't realize was that my baby's stomach was only the size of a cherry in those early days, and I didn't need to help my body bring on my milk faster. By day three, their tummy grows to the size of a walnut, and by the end of the first week, it's as big as an apricot. The best way to know if your baby is getting enough milk is to count wet diapers, monitor weight gain, and listen for swallowing sounds during feeding. To help boost my supply, I tried everything short of a rain dance:

- Staying hydrated – drinking two to three litres of water per day.
- Drinking electrolyte drinks every day.
- Adding oatmeal into your daily routine. I would have a big bowl of cooked oatmeal each morning and added oatmeal granola bars to my snack bag.
- Adding flaxseed to smoothies, oatmeal or baking.
- Adding brewers' yeast to smoothies or in baking.

Over Supply Being an over-supplier sounds like a dream, right? Well, let me tell you, it's like winning the lottery and finding out it's all in pennies. It's uncomfortable and tricky to manage. In the early days, I was feeding my baby from both breasts each session. This method turned me into a milk factory on overdrive. A baby gets both foremilk, which is watery and hydrating, and hindmilk, which is rich, and calorie packed when they feed from the breast. By offering both breasts he was not only gaining weight like a sumo wrestler at a buffet, but I was also telling my body to keep producing more and more.

To manage my oversupply, I was directed to nurse from only one breast per feed, offering that breast for a two-hour window.

After two hours, I switched to the opposite side. This method taught my body to chill out on the milk production. Here are a few things that helped me regulate my supply:

- **Peppermint tea** – Peppermint can lower milk supply. I chewed gum, used extracts, and drank tea like I was preparing for a British tea party. Steeping two tea bags in a large mug twice a day for three days worked best for me.
- **Allergy medication** – certain types of allergy medication is also known to lower milk supply. When I was struggling with blocked ducts my Lactation Consultant prescribed me to take one capsule a day for three days. This method didn't work as we had hoped, and I had to scale up the medication.
- **Decongestants** – Some decongestants can help reduce milk supply. Taking a capsule every twelve hours for two to three days turned out to be my secret weapon. It worked so well that I had to repeat it when my little guy started sleeping through the night, and I woke up feeling like a dairy cow that missed morning milking.

Overactive Letdown: Imagine trying to drink from a fire hose—that's what an overactive letdown feels like for a baby. My milk flowed faster than a river after a heavy rain, leaving my poor baby choking and sputtering. It was frustrating for both of us, but I learned a few tricks to manage when we nursed.

Feeding in a laid-back position, where I reclined slightly and let my baby nurse on top of me, helped to slow the flow. It felt like we were practicing baby yoga, but it worked. Taking frequent breaks to burp my baby also made a huge difference. Some mothers swear by pumping a little before each feed to control the flow, but given my status as an overproducer, my lactation consultant advised against it—lest I turn my kitchen into a dairy processing plant.

Teething: Ah, teething—a joyous milestone that can turn your sweet cherub into a tiny, over eager piranha. Most babies begin teething between four to seven months, but some overachievers start as early as three months. Others may take their sweet time and not start until closer to one year. Teething is a normal part of babyhood and can come with a host of delightful symptoms:

- **Excessive biting**: When your little one bites during nursing, it's best to gently remove them from the breast and firmly say "No." Try nursing again, but if the biting continues, it's time to call it quits for that session. They might need a reminder that your nipple is not a chew toy. Offering a teething toy can sometimes help them satisfy their urge to gnaw before trying to nurse again.
- **Wanting to suck at the breast more**: You may find that your baby wants to stay latched on like a barnacle. (This is where the nickname that my husband and I used had come from!) As long as they're actively nursing, they can't bite. But watch for cues that they're full or starting to play around—because nobody wants to be a teething toy.
- **Change in appetite and feeding schedule**: The pain and discomfort of teething can make babies less interested in feeding. The pressure on their gums can make sucking painful, so they might refuse the breast more often. You may see them starting and stopping more frequently, showing signs of discomfort like crying, fussing, or pulling away. Patience and a sense of humor go a long way during this phase. And maybe a teething toy or two!

Thrush: a yeast infection in the baby's mouth and on the mother's nipples, can cause significant discomfort. I was lucky enough to dodge the thrush bullet, but if we had encountered it, we would have been armed with antifungal medication. Some mothers use a vinegar and water solution to wipe the nipples after each feeding, which sounds like a recipe for making a sour face.

To keep things clean, I maintained a strict hygiene routine with my breast pump parts. I even went so far as to using separate cleaning brushes, because who wants spaghetti sauce residue on their pump flanges? I also showered daily, expressed milk, and used nipple cream whenever I thought my nipples looked or felt dry or irritated. Changing my nursing tank twice a day, thought maybe not necessary, was something I did as well. I wanted to make sure my nipples and breasts were always kept clean and sweat free. As my baby grew and began using pacifiers and toys, I became the sterilizing queen, ensuring that anything that hit the floor or ended up in the dog's mouth got washed. My baby's mouth was not a dog toy storage facility, after all.

Tongue and Lip Ties: a tongue-tie is a condition where the baby's tongue is restricted by a tight frenulum and a lip tie is a condition in which the piece of tissue that connects the upper lip to the upper gums, called the labial frenulum, is unusually tight, thick, or short. Both conditions can restrict the movement of the tongue and upper lip, making it difficult for a baby to latch properly during breastfeeding. If you suspect your little baby has a tongue or a lip tie it is best to have a lactation consultant or medical professional assess them. Thankfully my son did not have either of these conditions. Based on the input from the other mothers in the online support group I was a part of, it is fairly common for a baby to have one of these concerns.

Navigating my way through the common breastfeeding issues was certainly a challenge, but with the right support and resources we were able to manage, and it did not last for too long. Sore nipples, engorgement, latch issues, low or high milk supply, overactive letdown, blocked ducts, mastitis, thrush, and tongue and lip ties are all common hurdles that many mothers face. Remember that you are not alone, and seeking help from lactation consultants, healthcare providers, and support groups can provide you with the guidance and encouragement needed. Each challenge you overcome is a step forward in your breastfeeding journey, bringing you closer to a fulfilling and rewarding experience. And hey, if all else fails, there's always chocolate (for you, not the baby).

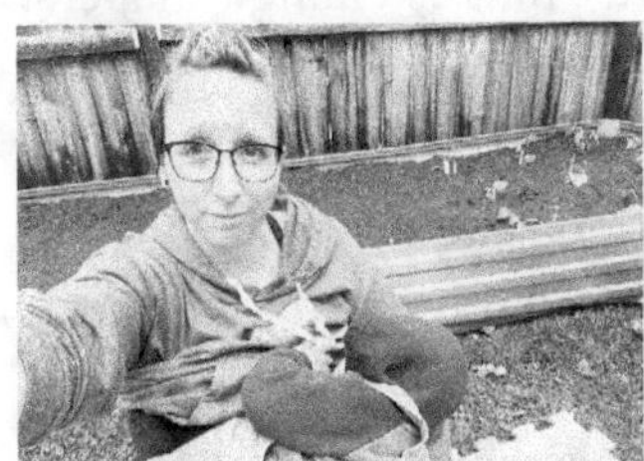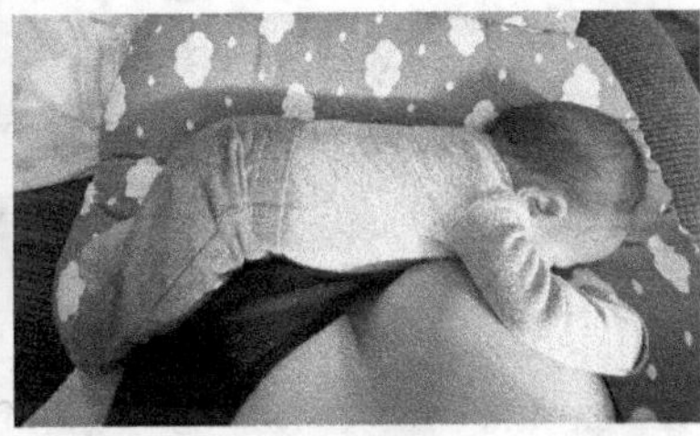

(Left) Stopped to feed while we were gardening in the backyard (Right) Nursing in the "Cross-cradle" position using the breast pillow

6

Finding Your Milk Groove

The Early Days: Establishing a Routine

Establishing a breastfeeding routine was a gradual process that evolved every couple of weeks. In the beginning, it felt like all I did was nurse, change diapers, and repeat. It was an endless cycle, morning and night, day after day. My family affectionately nicknamed me the "milk machine" and "baby bar." They joked I should start charging admission. Newborns need to feed frequently due to their small stomachs, often every 2-3 hours. While this constant demand was exhausting, it was essential for establishing a good milk supply and ensuring my baby received adequate nutrition.

Adjusting to Growth and Changes

As my son grew, the dynamics of breastfeeding evolved. The hospital initiated the practice of meticulously tracking feeding times, which breast was last used, and how long each feeding session lasted. I continued this practice at home, expanding the logs to include when vitamins were administered and detailed records of his napping patterns. I gradually transformed our living room into what I affectionately called 'mission control' for all things feeding-related. This comprehensive tracking became invaluable during consultations with our Lactation Consultant, providing a clear picture of our routine and helping us make precise adjustments as needed. Eventually, I transitioned from paper to a digital app on my phone, a move driven more by practicality than a desire for modernity—it was easier to update and less likely to get lost among the daily shuffle of household items.

Mastering the Transition

Around the nine-week mark, a significant milestone occurred—my son slept through the night for the first time, ten hours straight! It was so unexpected that I frequently checked on him to reassure myself that he was alright. Initially, I thought I would finally catch up on my own sleep. However, I soon found myself waking up from the pressure and discomfort of engorgement, sometimes overwhelmed to the point of tears.

To manage these challenging nights, I adjusted my pumping schedule with the guidance of my Lactation Consultant. Initially, I set an alarm to pump every two to three hours to relieve the pressure, which provided both physical and emotional relief. Gradually, I extended the intervals between pumping sessions to four to five hours. Once I adjusted to this new routine, my Lactation Consultant advised me to pump only until my breasts felt soft, rather than emptying them completely. This strategy was crucial as it taught my body not to overproduce or rapidly replace the milk that was expressed, helping to balance my milk supply with my son's changing needs. This adjustment allowed me to better align my pumping sessions with his natural waking hours and made the nighttime disruptions more manageable.

Adjusting to Evening Routines

Amidst this transition, I realized the importance of carving out time for myself during the evenings amid the constant daily demands of motherhood. My husband was always there to help me in the evenings when he was home from work, taking over baby duties and engaging our son with playful interaction or soothing him to sleep. This invaluable support allowed me some much-needed personal time. However, I didn't always get the solitude I planned for. Often, I'd come out of the shower to find them both peeking around the corner of the bathroom door—baby in my husband's arms, with him playfully asking, "What's mummy doing?" These little moments, though unexpected, were always a delightful reminder of the joyous and bustling life we were building together.

In the early days, I often found myself eating while my baby nursed. This meant that I ate my dinner over the top of him while he was latched and lying within the feeding pillow. As he got older and began to recognize different foods, mealtime turned into a delicate balancing act. One memorable evening, while I was carefully balancing a turkey and cheese sandwich over him, he reached up and grabbed it, causing slices of turkey, cheese, and bread to tumble down over both of us. He looked up at me with huge wide eyes in shock, but then we both burst into a fit of laughter, our laps covered in sandwich pieces. Despite these challenges, I have many fond memories of these shared moments, my son small and quiet, often falling asleep after feeding, leaving me to remain still until he woke up, and just watching him as time passed by.

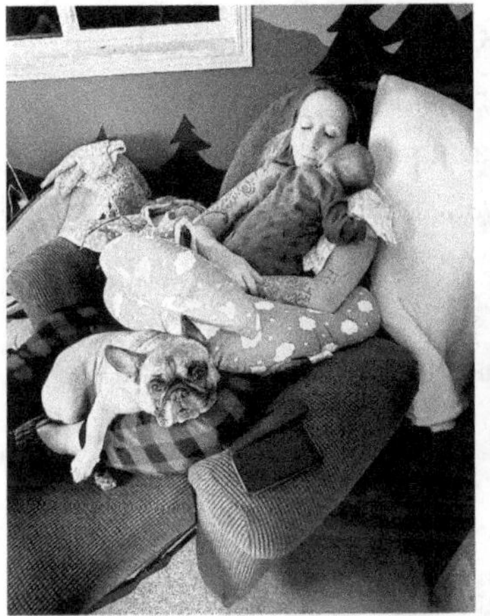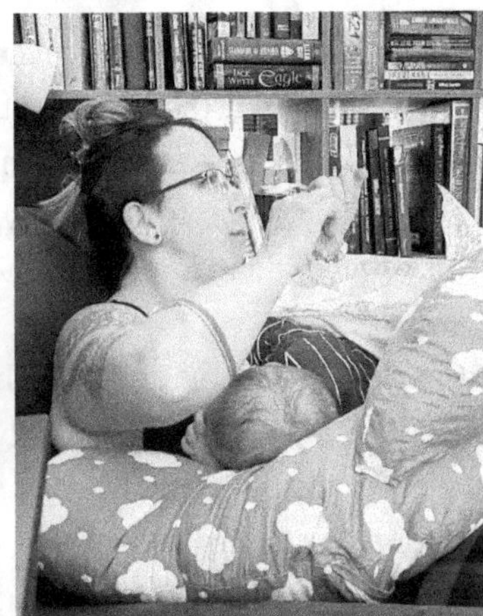

(Left) Personal space becomes non-existent when you are a mother
(Right) Enjoying dinner while my son nursed

Exploring Dietary Changes and Introducing Solids

As I settled into our refined routine, I discovered that certain foods I consumed affected my son's digestion. Foods like broccoli, cabbage, and spicy sauces were off the table. During my pregnancy, I was often too ill to eat much, but postpartum, my appetite surged. I felt like I couldn't eat enough, making it essential to consume high-protein meals, whole foods, and nutritious snacks. My go-to snacks included trail mix, peanut butter sandwiches, and Greek yogurt smoothies. I also began making a daily protein shake to boost my intake, which was like mixing a magic potion that kept me going (always check with your doctor before taking any supplements).

When my son was around five months old, we began introducing solids. He showed early interest, mimicking our eating actions with his toy cups, which was his version of 'fine dining.' This new stage was overwhelming initially as I balanced breastfeeding with solid food introductions, mindful of common allergens and his reactions. As he began consuming more solids, he naturally breastfed less. It was a bit like negotiating with a tiny but very determined CEO about his meal plan.

By paying close attention to his habits and maintaining a flexible schedule, we adapted smoothly to each new phase. Listening closely to my body and his cues, and continually seeking advice from my Lactation Consultant, ensured that our breastfeeding journey was effective, fulfilling, and enjoyable. This attentive and adaptive approach was the key to finding our milk groove, with a few laughs along the way.

7

Boobs in the Wild: Breastfeeding on the Go

Getting Equipped for the Milk Mission

Preparing to breastfeed in public is like packing for an expedition—knowing your tools and terrain is key. Learn about local laws that protect your right to nurse anywhere you're allowed to be. My nursing cover was my shield, and the different feeding positions were my strategies. Initially using a basic receiving blanket was like bringing a knife to a gunfight—it was too small, easily shifted, and I couldn't see his face or confirm his latch. Upgrading to a sturdy nursing cover was like switching to a Swiss army knife, offering me both privacy and peace of mind. What I found worked best for us was to get a rhythm down at home first, knowing which positions worked best and practicing using the nursing cover.

First-Time Jitters: Baby's First Public Snack

The initial days of venturing into public breastfeeding were filled with trepidation. Each time I considered nursing outside the safety of our home, I felt a twinge of anxiety. This nervousness was rooted not just in the physical exposure but in the vulnerability, it invited from the world around me. My shyness and embarrassment about breastfeeding in public initially led me to seek the confined privacy of our vehicle—a cramped but controlled environment where I could avoid the prying eyes and potential judgment of strangers.

This was also complicated by my fear of confrontation. I was acutely aware of the varied opinions on public breastfeeding, and the thought of facing disapproval or outright criticism was daunting. However, the logistical challenges of retreating to our car, compounded by the bitter cold of a Canadian winter, quickly highlighted the impracticality of my approach.

On one particularly challenging day, huddled in the backseat of the vehicle with my son fussing and the cold biting, I reached a turning point. I asked myself, "If everyone else can snack in public, why can't my baby?" That moment was a revelation. I realized I was allowing my fear of others' opinions to overshadow my baby's needs. This was my call to action. It wasn't just about feeding my baby—it was about asserting our right to do so as naturally and freely as anyone else would eat.

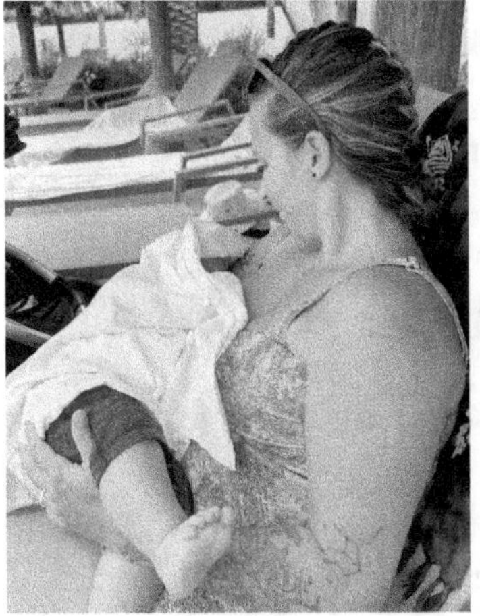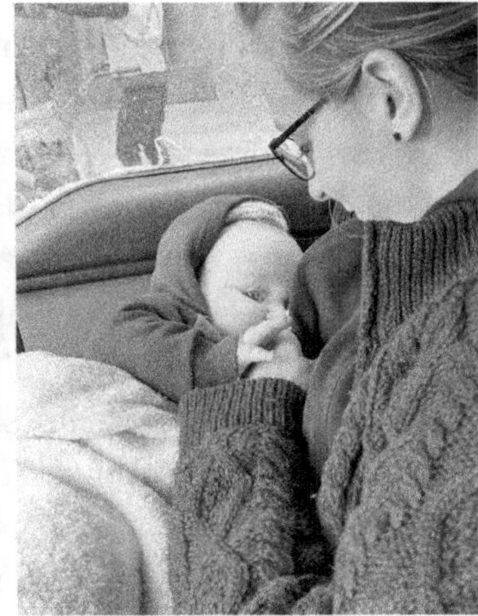

(Left) Breastfeeding pool-side while on vacation (Right) Feeding my son in the vehicle

Public Debut and Confidence Crusade

The real game-changer was during an outing at a shopping mall. Tucked in a corner with my husband, I nursed under a cover. No one seemed to notice, and spotting another mother doing the same reinforced my confidence. I remember glancing over at her, both of us giving each other a small, knowing nod. It was like a secret handshake of the breastfeeding world, and it filled me with a sense of pride that I could do that too. I wasn't just feeding my baby; I was part of a community standing up for our children's needs.

This shared moment shifted my perspective on motherhood and breastfeeding. What I once found uncomfortable turned into a proud public declaration of nurturing. The mall was no longer a place of anxiety but a stage for my newfound confidence. I realized I was not alone; there were other mothers just like me, following a similar journey.

From that point forward, I confidently nursed in a variety of locations. Mall benches became my nursing throne, restaurant booths my feeding stations, sunny park spots my serene breastfeeding oasis, and even crowded airplanes my high-altitude nursing lounges. With each new place, I felt more empowered, no longer feeling like I had to hide away. Turning every outing into an opportunity to normalize breastfeeding and show the world that feeding our babies is a beautiful, natural part of life. It was liberating to no longer feel confined to my home or the backseat of my car. Instead, I embraced the world with my baby in tow, ready to feed him whenever and wherever he needed.

The Convenience Factor

The convenience of breastfeeding truly is unmatched! The ability to pause and feed the baby wherever and whenever he needed was incredibly liberating. All it took was a simple cradle and cover, and voilà—my baby was content, and we could carry on with our day. This simplicity transformed our outings from potential stress-fests into smooth, manageable adventures.

Breastfeeding allowed me to be spontaneous and flexible. Whether we were out shopping, visiting friends, or enjoying a day at the park, I never had to worry about whether I had packed enough bottles or if there would be a place to warm them up. Instead of searching for the nearest microwave or asking for hot water at a restaurant, I could just find a quiet spot, settle in, and nurse my baby. I didn't have to lug around a cooler or worry about sterilizing bottles on the go. My body provided the perfect, warm, ready-to-serve meal every time. It was like having a magical, self-replenishing snack bar right there with me.

This ease of feeding made me deeply empathize with formula-feeding mothers who had to carry bottles, find facilities to warm them, and plan meticulously to ensure they were prepared for their baby's hunger. Watching them juggle all those supplies while keeping an eye on the clock made me appreciate the straightforwardness of breastfeeding even more. I realized just how many logistical hurdles were eliminated for me, making life on the go much simpler.

This convenience also extended to nighttime feedings. I didn't have to stumble to the kitchen half-asleep to prepare a bottle. I could simply lift my baby from his crib and nurse him, allowing us both to drift back to sleep more easily. This ease of nighttime nursing helped us both get more rest and made the whole experience less stressful.

The Mile High Milk Club

Flying with my baby introduced new challenges but also showcased the benefits of nursing-friendly clothing. Alongside my trusty nursing tanks, I found a hooded sweatshirt with cleverly concealed zippers, which allowed easy access without drawing attention. This attire proved invaluable in the tight confines of an airplane seat, letting me nurse discreetly and comfortably without the hassle of maneuvering a nursing cover with one hand while holding my baby in the other. My first solo flight with my son when he was four months old went far smoother than anticipated, thanks to these preparations. He nursed and slept through the entire journey, much to the amazement of the flight attendants who couldn't believe how calm a four-month-old could be on a flight.

The second trip I took with my son, when he was six months old and much more active, brought new adventures and mishaps. Thankfully for this adventure away we had my husband in tow.

During this flight, no sooner had we boarded the aircraft and just about to taxi away from the gate, my son surprised us with a massive diaper blowout! Trying to get him cleaned up and changed within the absurdly tiny airplane bathrooms was a real ordeal, especially when I discovered that not every bathroom was equipped with a baby change table. This "uh-oh" moment proved far more challenging than nursing and taught us valuable lessons for future travels. Ironically, it was his comfort and quiet I had worried about most! Once we were up in the air, despite the earlier chaos, he nursed for the remainder of the flight, which kept him calm and settled.

We took our third trip when he was eight months old, and by this point he was an experienced flyer, nursing on and off right from take off through to landing. It was incredibly convenient to be able to feed him on demand without worrying about preparing bottles or warming them up. We even shared a row with another mother who was juggling three premade formula bottles for her baby, who was just a month younger than our son, a reminder of how fortunate I felt to avoid that extra stress. Her experience, contrasting with mine, reinforced the benefits of breastfeeding on the go, even in challenging environments like an airplane.

The Good, the Bad, and the Snuggly

Despite overwhelmingly positive experiences, there was one memorable dinner at a family-friendly restaurant that felt more like an exhibition than a meal. It was a cold Canadian winter evening, with temperatures around -40°C, making it impractical to nurse in our vehicle. As I settled into the booth and started feeding my son under my cover while trying to enjoy my dinner, a neighboring table of onlookers grimaced as if they'd encountered something deeply unpleasant. They made me feel like the main attraction, glaring and whispering under their breaths. It made me feel incredibly uncomfortable, but we avoided confrontation as they kept their words to themselves. I focused on my baby and my food, trying to act like I didn't notice them. What else could I do? I didn't have a bottle with us, and my son was hungry and crying. I focused on my baby's needs, reminding myself of my rights and the essential nature of what I was doing. Despite their stares, I continued to nurse, committed to providing for my son.

8

Balancing Bottles and Briefcases

C hoosing the right kind of pump is important, especially when making the decision to return to work and continue breastfeeding. While a hand pump can work, investing in a high-quality rechargeable battery powered pump allows you to express milk from both breasts simultaneously, saving time and maintaining supply. Be sure to have breast pump wipes or cleaner in your bag to keep all the parts clean. Some mothers find it helpful to store their breast pump parts in the refrigerator to minimize cleaning during the workday. Just imagine explaining that to your co-workers: "No, that's not a science experiment, just my breast pump parts chilling next to your lunch!"

Claiming Your Space

Before you start pumping at work, it's essential to familiarize yourself with your workplace rights regarding breastfeeding. Many countries have laws that protect breastfeeding mothers, ensuring they provide a clean and private space (that is not a bathroom) for pumping. Discussing these needs with your employer before returning to work helps ensure that everyone is on the same page and prevents any potential miscommunication.

When I was preparing to return to work, I scheduled a meeting with my HR department to discuss my needs. I wanted to make sure I had a designated space that was comfortable and private. Fortunately, my employer was very understanding and provided a small, unused office for me to pump in. Knowing I had a safe and private space at work where I could pump without interruption gave me peace of mind and helped me focus better during the day.

It's also helpful to create a pumping schedule that aligns with your workday. Communicate this schedule with your team if necessary, so they understand when you'll be unavailable. This transparency can help avoid any misunderstandings and ensures you can pump consistently, maintaining your milk supply without added stress.

Bottle Bootcamp

Introducing a bottle to your baby before returning to work can help ensure a smooth transition. Timing is key—wait until breastfeeding is well-established, typically around 4-6 weeks, to avoid nipple confusion. Start by choosing a slow-flow nipple that mimics the flow of breastfeeding to make the transition easier for your baby.

The introduction process can be tricky. Initially, have someone else offer the bottle, as your baby associates you with breastfeeding and may refuse the bottle from you. This is a great opportunity for your partner or another caregiver to bond with the baby. Start with small amounts of breast milk in the bottle and gradually increase as your baby becomes more comfortable.

Patience is essential during this phase. Some babies take

to the bottle immediately, while others may need more time. You might find yourself going through a small mountain of rejected bottles before finding the right one that your baby likes. Experiment with different bottle brands and nipple shapes if needed, and don't get discouraged if it takes a while.

Milk Stash Mastery

Once you begin pumping at work, it's essential to have a way to keep the milk cold and fresh. If your workplace has a refrigerator, store the milk in bottles or breast milk storage bags, and label each container with the date and time it was collected.

Pro tip: Label your milk so that nobody accidentally uses it for their coffee. Imagine the horror of someone unknowingly creating a "lactation latte"! I always kept the milk and pump parts in a lunch bag, which served as a discreet barrier. This way, others wouldn't open the fridge and be greeted by a display of breast milk bottles mingling with their lunches.

To transport the milk home at the end of each day, I would use the lunch bag with some ice packs. This simple yet effective method ensured that the milk stayed cool and safe during the commute. Once home, the milk would either go into the fridge or the freezer, depending on our needs for the next few days.

It's different in each country, so be sure to check what's recommended where you live. The guidelines for storing breast milk vary, but generally, breast milk can be kept at room temperature for up to four hours, in the fridge for up to four days, and in the freezer for up to six months (or up to a year in some types of freezers). Always ensure that the milk is properly stored immediately after pumping. The sight of my growing milk stash in the freezer was incredibly satisfying—a testament to my dedication and a handy backup for days when I might need a break.

Organizing the milk stash became a fun little project. I used a simple first-in, first-out system to ensure that the oldest milk got used up first, preventing waste. Some mothers even invest in special breast milk storage organizers that fit into your freezer like a drawer. This keeps everything neat and makes grabbing the oldest bag of milk a breeze.

Pump Like a Pro

Maintaining your milk supply when going back to work is very important. The strategies you use may depend on when you return to work. If you go back earlier, adhering to a regular pumping schedule is crucial. Think of it as setting your own internal clock to "milk o'clock." If you are returning to work after a year of maternity leave, you may not need to pump as often, as your body may have already self-regulated to feed less frequently. You might even have started the weaning process. This is different for all mothers, and they need to do what is best for them and their baby. Some might find that their little one is more interested in solid foods than a liquid diet, while others may still prefer the comfort of nursing.

Regular and consistent pumping is key. It is best to try and pump at the same times each day. This helps maintain your milk supply and creates a routine that your body can rely on. You might need to boost your production with lactation-boosting foods like oatmeal or lactation cookies. And try not to stress—easier said than done, I know. Stress can impact milk supply, so find ways to relax while pumping. Listen to music, look at photos of your baby, or practice deep breathing. Maybe throw in a podcast or two—true crime, anyone? Nothing like a little mystery to pass the time while you're hooked up to a machine!

Home Sweet Home

Continue breastfeeding at home to maintain your supply and bond with your baby. Nursing in the morning, evening, and during the night can help sustain milk production. The transition back to work can be emotionally challenging, so stay connected with your baby through frequent feedings when you're together, and seek support from family, friends, or a breastfeeding support group. Remember, you're not alone in this – think of it as joining an elite club of multitasking supermoms who can handle anything, from board meetings to midnight feedings.

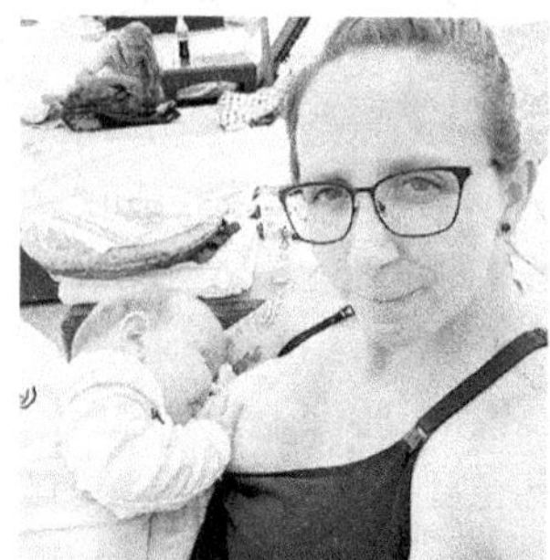
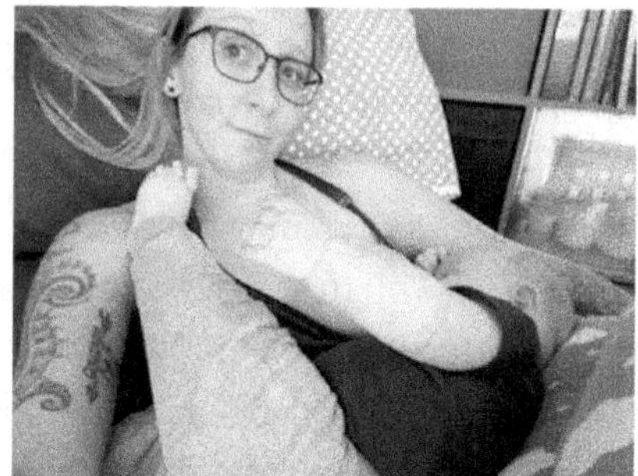

(Left) Nursing my son while on an outdoor adventure (Right) Nursing became more of a challenge the bigger and more active my son got

9

Milk, Love, and Lullabies: Bonding Through Breastfeeding

The Love Hormone

Breastfeeding is not just about providing nutrition; it's also a deeply emotional experience that fosters a unique bond between mother and baby. Holding my baby close, skin-to-skin, and gazing into his eyes during feedings created a powerful connection. These moments of closeness were some of the most profound and rewarding aspects of motherhood. Imagine my surprise when I realized my baby already had me wrapped around his tiny, milk-drunk fingers.

The oxytocin released during breastfeeding, often referred to as the "love hormone," played a significant role in strengthening this bond. This hormone helps with milk letdown and promotes feelings of love and attachment. Every time my baby latched on, it was like a wave of calm and contentment washed over me, even if I had just been on the brink of a mini meltdown. The love hormone turned these feeding sessions into magical bonding moments, making the sleepless nights and endless diaper changes seem a little more manageable. Each feeding session became an opportunity to nurture my baby both physically and emotionally, reinforcing the strong bond we were building. It's like oxytocin was nature's little way of reminding me that amidst the chaos, there was this beautiful connection blooming between us.

Emotional Rollercoaster

While breastfeeding promotes the release of the 'love hormone,' it also comes with challenges such as postpartum depression and sleep deprivation. The postpartum period is a time of immense emotional change, marked by hormonal shifts and the relentless demands of caring for a newborn. I experienced moments of pure joy and love, but also feelings of overwhelming anxiety, anger, and sadness. Breastfeeding itself can be both a source of comfort and a trigger for emotional stress. The pressure to succeed, combined with the physical demands, sometimes left me feeling inadequate and "touched out."

By the end of the day, I was completely exhausted. Despite loving my baby more than anything, I felt like I had no more capacity to give. The constant need for physical contact and attention from my baby drained me. I often felt guilty because, while I adored my child, I couldn't handle anyone else needing my attention—whether physical or emotional. There were moments when I felt like I had become a human pacifier, and the only thing missing was a "Do Not Disturb" sign around my neck.

In those early postpartum days, it was hard to even want to show my partner affection. The idea of more touch, even a loving hug or a gentle caress, felt overwhelming. I needed space to recharge, but the demands of a newborn rarely allowed it. My husband, understanding yet occasionally feeling sidelined, had to adjust to the new dynamics of our relationship. This period tested our patience and communication, highlighting the need for understanding and support.

It was important for me to acknowledge these feelings and seek support when needed. Talking to my husband, other mothers, and joining support groups provided a sense of solidarity and relief. Consulting with medical professionals helped me navigate the emotional challenges of the postpartum period. They reassured me that feeling "touched out" was a common experience among new mothers and that taking care of my emotional well-being was just as important as caring for my baby.

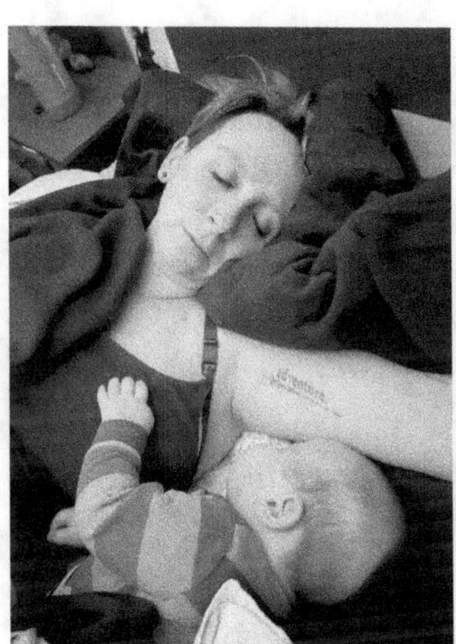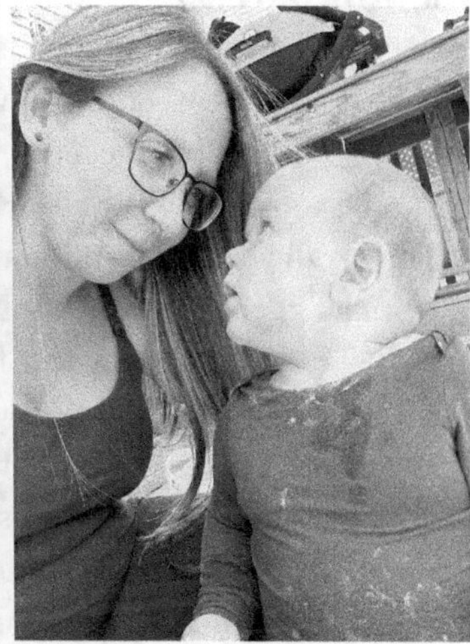

(Left) Both mum and son sleeping (Right) A proud mum and son, post snack

Skin-to-Skin Superpowers

I made it a point to incorporate skin-to-skin time into our

daily routine, not just during feedings but also during moments of calm and rest even as he got older. This practice helped soothe my son, making him feel secure and loved, and reinforced the strong emotional connection we were building. It also helped me to feel at ease and focus on something other than the post partum depression.

When I faced difficulties, such as latch issues or low milk supply, I sometimes felt frustrated and anxious. It was necessary for me to seek help and support, and my lactation consultant was a superhero in disguise. She always seemed to have the perfect advice or trick up her sleeve to get us back on track.

The Night Owl Club

One of the most challenging aspects of the early days of motherhood is sleep deprivation. Newborns need to feed frequently, including throughout the night, which means interrupted sleep for both mother and baby. The lack of continuous sleep took a toll on my physical and emotional well-being.

To manage sleep deprivation, I tried to rest whenever my baby slept, even if it was just for short naps. This of course was easier said than done. It was the time that my son was sleeping that I used to catch up on showering and spending time with my four-legged house mates. Co-sleeping in a safe manner and setting up a comfortable nursing station by the bed made nighttime feedings more manageable. My husband's support was valuable during this time; he helped with diaper changes and comforting the baby, allowing me to focus on breastfeeding and getting some rest. He also stepped up and handled much of the household work that had to take a back seat when I brought the baby home, helping to prepare and cook meals and household chores. He became the master chef of the quickest, most nutritious meals—bless him.

Understanding that sleep deprivation is a temporary phase helped me cope better. As my baby grew and his feeding patterns became more regular, my sleep gradually improved. Until that happened, I found solace in the fact that we were both in this sleepless journey together, like two little night owls navigating the darkness.

Melodies and Memories

Every nursing session was an opportunity to celebrate the bond between my baby and me. These moments of closeness, love, and connection were priceless. The act of nurturing my baby through breastfeeding became a cherished part of our daily routine, creating lasting memories and strengthening our relationship.

And let's not forget the countless hours I spent researching and memorizing lullabies because, apparently, I couldn't remember a single word from the ones I heard as a child. It turns out, "Twinkle, Twinkle, Little Star" has more than one verse—who knew? I found myself singing "The Itsy-Bitsy Spider" on repeat until it became my new jam. I even made up a few verses of my own to keep things interesting. The soundtrack of our breastfeeding journey was a mix of classic lullabies and my own off-key creations, but my baby didn't seem to mind one bit.

Breastfeeding is a journey that encompasses much more than just providing nutrition. It is a powerful tool for bonding and emotional connection between mother and baby. Navigating the emotional aspects, including postpartum challenges and sleep deprivation, requires patience, support, and self-care. By embracing the emotional journey of breastfeeding, I was able to build a strong and loving bond with my baby, enriching our lives in ways that went beyond the physical benefits of breast milk.

And in the end, those late-night feedings and lullaby sessions became some of our most treasured times together. There's something magical about those quiet, sleepy moments when the world feels like it's just you and your little one, sharing secrets and songs under the soft glow of a nightlight. These were the moments that made the exhaustion and challenges worthwhile, creating memories that I will carry with me always.

10

From Milk to Meals: Our Weaning Journey

As my son and I journeyed together through the transition from exclusive breastfeeding to introducing solid foods began sooner than anticipated. This significant milestone brought a complex mix of emotions, from pride and accomplishment to nostalgia and a touch of sadness. Our weaning process, deeply personal like every step of our breastfeeding adventure, reflects our unique bond and the baby-led weaning path we embraced.

The World of Baby-Led Weaning

Around five months, my son's curiosity about the world of flavors began to blossom. He would eagerly reach for my plate, his wide eyes following every motion of my fork and spoon, mimicking my chewing with an open, expectant mouth. After consulting with our doctor and ensuring he was ready, we decided to dive into the world of baby-led weaning. This approach allowed him to explore a variety of foods at his own pace, promoting his independence and helping him learn to regulate his intake based on fullness. It also aimed to ward off picky eating while enhancing his motor skills through the handling of different food shapes and sizes.

The early stages of introducing solids were an absolute delight, marked by my son's infectious enthusiasm for new tastes and textures. Each mealtime was an exciting exploration. I started with easy-to-handle soft fruits and vegetables like bananas, strawberries, and melon. Watching his reactions—varied facial expressions ranging from joy to cautious skepticism—was profoundly endearing.

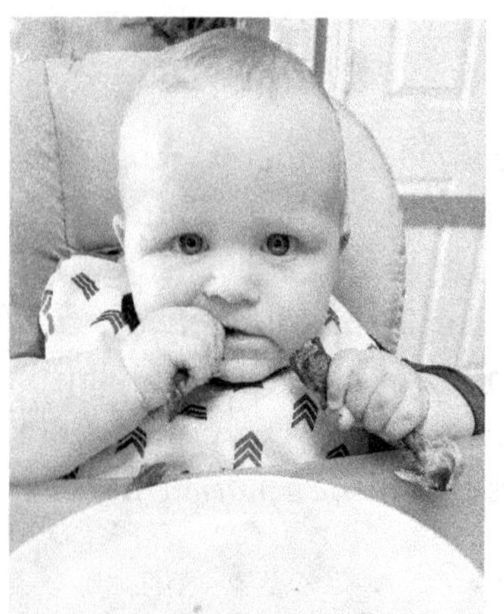 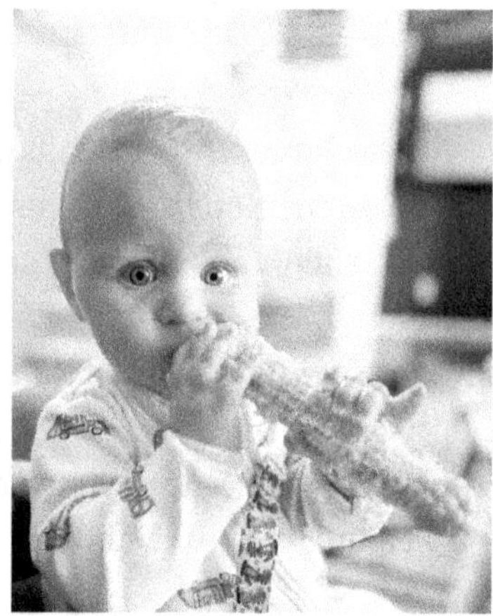

(Left) Enjoying a chicken drumstick (Right) Doing his best to eat corn on the cob

Mealtime Mayhem and Joy

As he grew more adventurous, I began mirroring my meals in his dishes, simplifying meal preparation and encouraging a shared family dining experience. This not only reduced the workload but also integrated him more fully into our mealtime rituals. His clear preference for proteins like chicken drumsticks and pork chops soon became apparent, revealing his little carnivorous inclinations.

With this exploration, however, came the inevitable chaos of mealtime messes. Each feeding was like inviting a tiny food critic to a finger-painting session where colorful smears of fruits and vegetables adorned the high chair, the floor, and sometimes even the walls. These moments, though messy, were filled with laughter and learning, reminding us that a little disorder is just part of the process. Our two house hippo's (Ollie and Piggy, our French bulldogs) reveled in the mess that always followed a meal time!

Embracing the Weaning Process

As our journey progressed to his first birthday and beyond, the balance between breastfeeding and solid foods naturally shifted. Nursing sessions gradually decreased, mainly surrounding nap times and bedtime—moments that continued to comfort him and provide a reassuring closeness in our day.

Despite the joys, the path wasn't without its bumps. Days when he would refuse nearly every solid offered or seemed to want to nurse endlessly, often driven by teething discomfort or the common colds of early childhood, were challenging. These fluctuations required patience and understanding, as they reminded me of the ongoing need for flexibility in our weaning process. During the days he was less interested in nursing, I managed any pending engorgement by using ice packs and wearing tighter clothing such as sports bras and snug tank tops. This approach, much like in the early days of breastfeeding, helped maintain comfort and gradually reduce my milk supply. I also incorporated peppermint tea into my morning routine, which aided in comfortably managing the milk reduction.

By then, he was naturally nursing less, and with the combination of daycare, work, and a full diet, it felt like the right time to end. Though bittersweet, this transition marked a natural progression in his growth. Weaning is far more than just the cessation of breastfeeding; it's a continuation of nurturing, a way to sustain the bond formed through countless hours of closeness. As we moved towards completely weaning, our nursing sessions dwindled down to tender moments filled with mixed emotions—each one a gentle step towards a new kind of independence.

This transition, though bittersweet, was also a celebration of growth, marked by the loving routines we established and the new ways we found to connect beyond breastfeeding. It was a natural progression, one that echoed the inevitable changes and developments in our lives. Should I be blessed with another child, I look forward to possibly revisiting this beautiful aspect of motherhood, armed with the knowledge and experiences from this invaluable chapter in our lives. As we closed this chapter, I felt a profound sense of gratitude for the journey and the bond that, though transformed, would always remain a fundamental part of us.

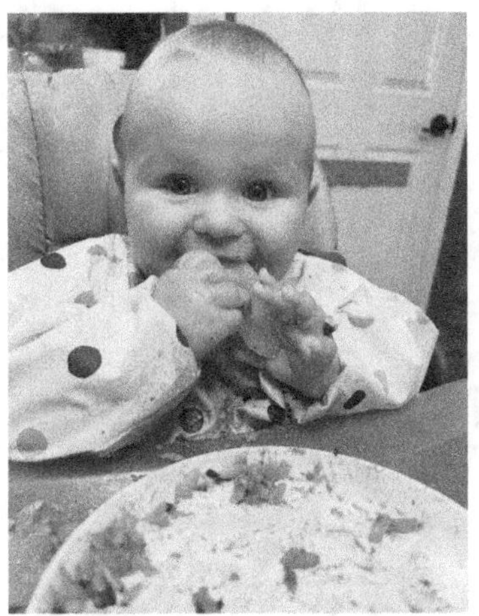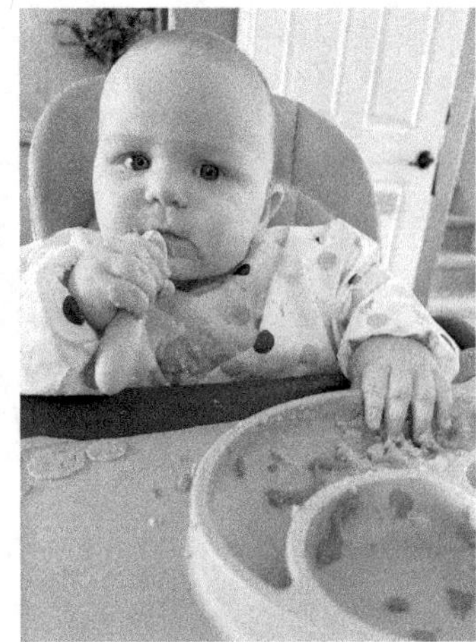

(Left) Baby-led weaning sure is messy! (Right) Showing his independence by feeding himself

11

What I've Learned and Wish I Knew

Reflecting on my journey, I marvel at the profound connection it fostered between my son and me. Breastfeeding is more than just nourishment; it is an intimate dance, a language of love, comfort, and security. As I look back on my own experience, I am filled with a mixture of emotions—pride, joy, frustration, and, above all, gratitude. By sharing my reflections and advice, I hope to offer support and encouragement to other mothers on this remarkable journey.

A Steep Learning Curve

From the very beginning, breastfeeding presented itself as a combination of natural and learned experiences. The early days were marked by a steep learning curve, filled with moments of doubt and worry. I constantly questioned whether I was producing enough milk, if the latch was correct, and whether the pain I felt was normal. It was a time of immense vulnerability, but also a time of incredible bonding. I felt like I was back in school, trying to ace the most important test of my life without any doing any studying beforehand.

One of the most valuable pieces of advice I can offer is to be patient with yourself and your baby. Breastfeeding is a skill that both of you develop together. It requires time, practice, and sometimes, a lot of perseverance. In the beginning, feedings were frequent and unpredictable. There were sleepless nights and days that seemed to blur together. Yet, each nursing session was an opportunity to learn and grow together. With time, we found our rhythm. My baby's latch improved, my milk supply regulated to his needs, and the initial discomfort and worry faded away.

Support Squad

Seeking support is crucial. I cannot emphasize enough the importance of reaching out to a lactation consultant, joining breastfeeding support groups, and leaning on other mothers for advice and encouragement. There were times when I felt overwhelmed and unsure but talking to experienced medical professionals and fellow mothers provided me with reassurance and practical solutions. They helped me navigate challenges like engorgement, sore nipples, and the many growth spurts and regressions. Knowing that I was not alone in my struggles made a significant difference. It was like having a personal cheerleading squad, minus the pom-poms.

Flexibility

Flexibility is another key aspect of successful breastfeeding. While it's beneficial to have a routine, it's equally important to adapt to your baby's needs. I found this to be an interesting struggle as I have always been the kind of individual who likes to plan and be prepared, but I found that babies don't have this on their agenda at all. There were days when my baby wanted to nurse constantly and others when he was more content between feedings. Listening to his cues and being responsive helped us both feel more at ease. I learned to trust my instincts and my body's ability to provide what he needed. Flexibility in nursing is a lot like yoga—sometimes you have to bend and stretch in ways you never thought possible.

Breastfeeding in Public

Breastfeeding in public was initially a daunting prospect. I worried about the judgement of others. However, as I gained confidence, I realized that feeding my baby was a natural and necessary act. I gained the confidence to feed anywhere, not always having to find a discreet place, just somewhere comfortable for the both of us. Using nursing covers and nursing clothing helped as well. As time had progressed, feeding in public just became part of our regular routine. It helped immensely that the judgement I was so afraid of was really nonexistent. I had found over time that many others had nursed their own babies or were familiar with it because of family members nursing. Many were very helpful and understanding. It turns out, people are more interested in their lattes than what's happening under my nursing cover.

Finding Joy

One of the unexpected joys of breastfeeding was the sense of accomplishment it brought. Knowing that I was providing my baby with the best possible nutrition and nurturing his growth was incredibly rewarding. Each successful feeding felt like a small victory. There were tough days, certainly, but there were also countless moments of pure contentment—watching my baby nurse peacefully, feeling the warmth of his tiny body against mine, and knowing that I was his source of comfort and sustenance. This is an experience that I miss to this very day and believe I will miss as the years progress.

Weaning

As my son grew, our journey evolved. Introducing solid foods and gradually weaning were new milestones that brought their own set of challenges and emotions. Weaning, in particular, was a bittersweet process. It marked the end of an era but also the beginning of new adventures. The exactment of trying new foods was fun for all of us and provided short term distractions away from nursing. Through it all, I learned to cherish each stage, knowing that these moments were fleeting and precious.

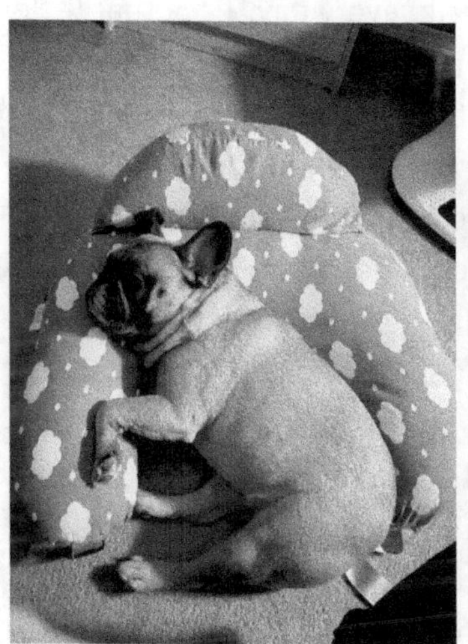
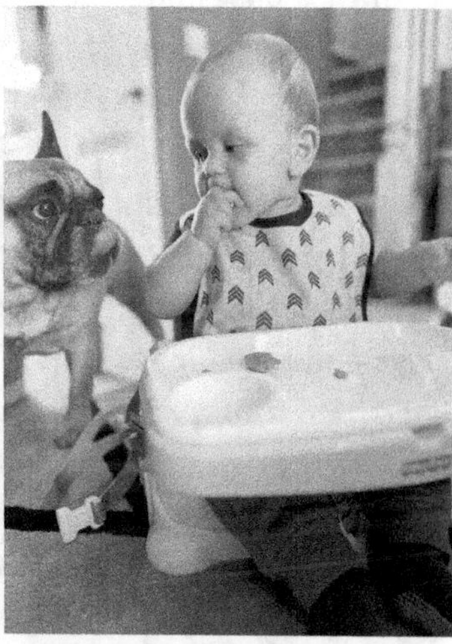

(Left) Breast pillows are not only comfy for a mother and baby, but furry friends too (Right) My boy sharing his cookies with our "house hippo"

Prioritizing Self Care

Often overlooked, is the aspect of self-care. It's vital to remember that taking care of yourself is just as important as caring for your little one. Breastfeeding is physically and emotionally demanding, so finding time for rest, relaxation, and activities that replenish your mind and spirit is crucial. This might mean taking a short walk, indulging in a favorite hobby, or simply allowing yourself a few moments of quiet each day. Ensuring that you are well-rested and emotionally balanced directly impacts your ability to nurture your baby effectively.

Making sure to be active during your post partum and healing days is the most beneficial thing, in my opinion, that you can do to help with post partum depression and anger. Get yourself out of the house and go for a walk, every day. Pack that little baby up in the stroller, grab a coffee or a bottle of water and get those two legs walking. Even it if it's just around the block! The sunshine and fresh air will help to clear your head, and it's a change of scenery from the same mundane walls of your house.

Fueling your body with healthy choices is another critical component. The quality of your diet influences your energy levels and the composition of your milk. Eating a balanced diet rich in fruits, vegetables, whole grains, and lean proteins provides the necessary nutrients to sustain both you and your baby. Staying hydrated is equally important. Make it a habit to drink water regularly, especially during and after nursing sessions. I was also incredibly thirsty while I was nursing—my thirst rivaled that of a marathon runner—and it was important to hydrate when I felt that way as it helped my body to produce more milk. By nourishing your body with wholesome foods and adequate hydration, you support your overall well-being and your nursing journey.

Trust your Instincts

Trusting your instincts is perhaps the most empowering advice I can offer. Trust yourself and trust your baby. You know your baby better than anyone else, and your intuition is a powerful guide. There will be moments when well-meaning advice from others may conflict with what feels right for you and your baby. In those times, trust yourself. You are the expert on your baby's needs, and your instincts will often lead you in the right direction. Embrace your inner confidence and believe in your ability to provide the best care for your child. The breastfeeding journey is unique to each pair, and there is no one right way to navigate it. Be kind to yourself, especially on the tough days. Seek support and don't hesitate to ask for help. Celebrate the small victories and be patient with the process. Remember that breastfeeding is not just about providing milk; it's about building a relationship and nurturing your baby with love and care.

Soak it All In

The tough days are going to feel like they will last forever, and you'll never adapt. The good days are often overshadowed by sleep deprivation and exhaustion. My advice to you: enjoy as much of this journey as you possibly can. It goes by so fast, and before you know it, your little one is not so little anymore. Blink, and they've gone from a sweet nursing infant to a toddler throwing their dinner back at you. The moments of bonding, the quiet times together, and even the challenging times all form a tapestry of experiences that you will cherish.

As my husband constantly reminded me, "It's all temporary." This means that even when the bad days feel endless, everything passes and evolves, and soon you'll be through it, onto the next stage. His words were a comforting reminder that the difficult phases are fleeting.

Soak it all in and treasure these fleeting moments. The struggles and triumphs alike are part of the beautiful journey of parenthood, creating memories you'll look back on with a smile.

Reflections

As I reflect on my breastfeeding journey, I am filled with a deep sense of gratitude and accomplishment. This experience has taught me about resilience, patience, and the profound bond between mother and child. To all the mothers embarking on or continuing this path, know that you are not alone. Every drop of milk, every sleepless night, and every quiet moment of connection with your baby is a testament to your strength and dedication. Cherish the small victories, trust your instincts, and soak in every precious moment. Remember, breastfeeding is not just about nourishment; it's about love, comfort, and creating lasting memories. Thank you for joining me on this journey. I hope my story has offered you insights, comfort, and encouragement. Embrace your unique journey with confidence and know that you are giving your baby a beautiful gift. Here's to all the mothers who navigate this incredible journey with grace, determination, and boundless love.

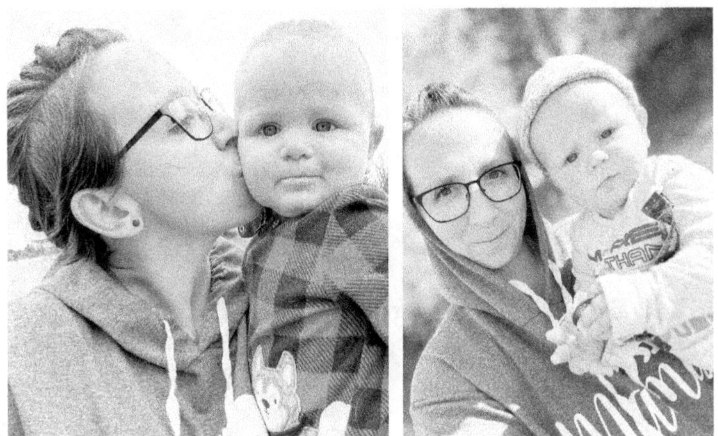

A proud mom and her son

12

Resources

1. Hospital Nurses at South Health Campus Hospital in Calgary, AB.
2. My Lactation Consultant and Family Physician.
3. Stanford Medicine. (2006). Hand expression of breastmilk. Stanford Medicine: Newborn Nursery. Retrieved June 28, 2024, from https://med.stanford.edu/newborns/professional-education/breastfeeding/hand-expressing-milk.html
4. Murkoff, H., & Mazel, S. (2008). What to expect when you're expecting: 4th edition. Workman Publishing.
5. Alberta Health Services. (2018). The Early Years: Healthy Parents, Healthy Children (Third printing) [Print].
6. What is Baby-Led Weaning? Benefits of BLW - Solid Starts. (n.d.). https://solidstarts.com/baby-led-weaning/

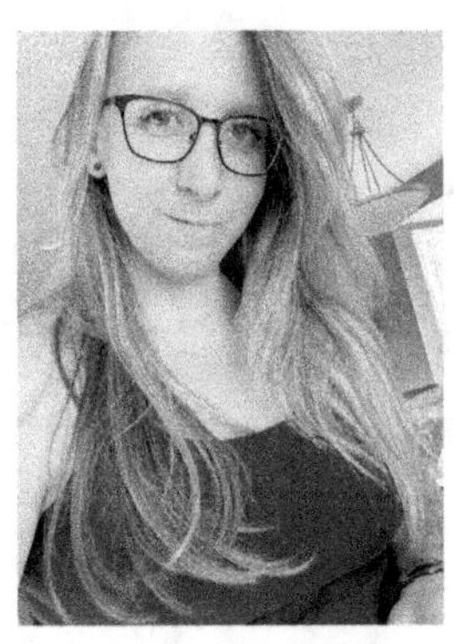

About the Author

Maddisson is a devoted wife and mother who lives with her husband, son and two French bulldogs near the Rocky Mountains in Alberta, Canada. She is an aspiring artist, who enjoys cooking nutritious meals, dirt biking, wood working and traveling to see her family.

You can connect with me on:

- https://www.instagram.com/hulmingbird
- https://www.tiktok.com/@hulmingbird